HEAD GAMES

Football's Concussion Crisis from the NFL to Youth Leagues

Christopher Nowinski

Introduction by Jesse Ventura, former high school football coach,
NFL commentator, and governor of Minnesota

D0057618

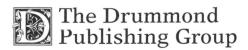

The Drummond
Publishing Group

The information and suggestions found in this book are designed to provide a re-source that may be useful in making informed choices about participation in sport-ing activities. The book is not intended to, and does not, provide medical advice, nor substitute for evaluation and treatment of any specific medical symptoms or conditions by a medical professional and should not be relied upon in any form or to any extent for that purpose. The author is not licensed to practice medicine nor physical or rehabilitational therapy of any form. Except as otherwise noted, the views expressed in the book are those of the author based upon his personal experi-ences, interviews of athletes, medical and therapeutic professionals and others con-nected to the topic, and his lay analysis of various medical studies and available data on the topics presented in the book. Each of the author and the publisher specifi-cally disclaim any liability or responsibility to any person for any decisions or actions taken in reliance on the information provided, or the views expressed, herein. Any person who has questions regarding a particular medical condition or symptoms similar to those described in this book is urged to consult a licensed physician expert in the field.

Copyright © 2007

THE DRUMMOND PUBLISHING GROUP
362 North Bedford St.
East Bridgewater, MA 02333

First Edition
10 9 8 7 6 5 4 3 2

Printed and bound in the UNITED STATES
ISBN: 1-59763-013-6
LIBRARY OF CONGRESS CONTROL NUMBER: 2006930723

To the players, young and old,
whose lives have been changed
forever by head injuries

Contents

Acknowledgments

I began writing and researching this book while recovering from a head injury. Few people would be able understand how much this book grew, and I grew, in the three years it took to complete. With that in mind, I owe an enormous debt of gratitude to the people that believed in me, supported me, and contributed to this work along the way, because I now realize there was never any way of knowing if I would recover enough to see this through.

First I'd like to thank my attorney and agent, Barbara Jones, for her tireless efforts.

I would like to thank Dr. Robert Cantu for his unwavering support and guidance throughout my research, Dr. Heechin Chae for his expertise and generosity, and all the other doctors mentioned in the text that took the time to educate me on this most complicated subject, and who are conducting the research shedding light on this dark area of knowledge.

So many people played a role in making this book happen. John Corcoran, Dave Fitzhenry, and everyone at Trinity Partners taught me the tools to perform this type of medical research and then gave me the professional freedom to do it. My editor, Gordon Laws, provided terrific advice and great passion for the project. Alan Schwarz and Ken Leiker, two very talented writers, went out of their way to help out a guy they hardly knew. Walter Norton Jr. not only kept me healthy and focused, but was a sounding board for ideas I had in the last three years. Melissa Panchuck's advice was indispensable.

I'd like to thank the WWE and the McMahon family for understanding and respecting my injury, and for sticking by me throughout this ordeal. It's been a joy to work with Gary Davis, Kate Cox, and Sue Aitchison in my new role there. I will also always be grateful to Head Coach Tim Murphy and everyone involved with the Harvard football program for the opportunity to play for the Crimson. This work should in no way reflect negatively on either the football program or the medical staff, both of which I hold in the highest regard.

I interviewed dozens of athletes and their families for this book, and I'd like to express my appreciation to every person that appears in the text and those who do not. It took courage to share their personal experiences, thoughts, and doubts.

I'd like to single out the following people who do not fit into one of the above categories for their counsel, assistance, or encouragement: Governor Jesse Ventura, Mick Foley, Billy Fairweather, Sal Paolantonio, Jeremy Schaap, Ruben Millor, Tina Cantu, Julius Bishop, Charles Wells, Sue Wells, Caroline Myss, Anthony Loscalzo, Jen Savage, Kate Taylor-Steeves, Barbara MacNeill, Aron Valevich, Tim Warner, Lisa Fenn, Brooke de Lench, Brian Daigle, Nick Fisher, Leslie Sandberg, SHAD, David Byer, Amy Matthews, Artie Clifford, Jennifer Phillips, and Beth Adams. If I forgot anyone, and I'm sure I did, you know why.

Finally, I'd like to thank my family. It was great to know I always had somewhere to go if I washed out.

Foreword

I am pleased to provide some opening words for this major work by Christopher Nowinski on a topic of long personal interest and research.

The head is unique in that its content, the brain, is largely incapable of regeneration. Thus, a brain injury takes on a singular importance. While today many parts of the body can be replaced either by artificial hardware or transplantation, the brain cannot be replaced.

Interest in and the published medical literature about the most mild of sports-related brain injuries, the cerebral concussion, has increased exponentially over the last decade. Once thought of as a transient impairment of brain function, we are now aware that concussion may lead to permanent neurological deficits and can end a sports career. The media has devoted extensive coverage to a number of prominent athletes who were forced to retire due to enduring symptoms following multiple cerebral concussions. Both the National Football League and National Hockey League are devoting time and money towards studying this problem.

It is obvious, given the potential serious consequences of especially multiple cerebral concussions, that prevention is paramount. Yet in many collision sports, even when played with proper technique, a cerebral concussion is an inherent risk of the sport. Furthermore, compounding the problem, in especially the helmeted sports, most mild concussions go unrecognized by sideline medical personnel.

In this book, Chris Nowinski in a personal, provocative, compelling, and authoritative manner affords the lay public comprehensive insight into sports-related concussion. I recommend this book ardently to every athlete of especially contact/collision sports and to their parents and family. Chris has compiled an encyclopedic resource on this topic that will not only enhance informed decisions by athletes and their families but also, with the knowledge contained in between these covers, afford safer participation. Furthermore, I hope and expect it will stimulate ever-increasing interest and needed critical study on this currently hotly debated topic.

ROBERT C. CANTU, M.A., M.D., F.A.C.S., F.A.C.S.M.

Chairman, Department of Surgery; Chief, Neurosurgery Service; and Director, Service Sports Medicine; Emerson Hospital, Concord, Massachusetts.

Adjunct Professor, Exercise and Sport Science University of North Carolina, Chapel Hill; Medical Director, National Center for Catastrophic Sports Injury Research Chapel Hill, North Carolina.

Co-Director, Neurological Sports Injury Center at Brigham and Women's Hospital, Boston, MA.

Neurosurgery Consultant, Boston College Eagles and Boston Cannon's Lacrosse teams.

Introduction

I have always enjoyed wrestling with difficult truths. I have confronted them in politics; I have confronted them in the military; and I now believe it is time to confront another difficult truth: that the concussion problem in football and other contact sports is far more serious than any of us want to believe, and it is time to do something about it.

You may know me from my time as the governor of Minnesota, as a professional wrestler, or as an actor, but before I was any of those things, I was a football player. I started in grade school, playing for five years, and then played three seasons for Theodore Roosevelt High School in Minneapolis, Minnesota, as a defensive end. I went on to play a year of service ball in the Navy while stationed in Subic Bay in the Philippines, and a year of junior college football upon returning to the States.

Since I stopped playing, I have remained an avid football fan and have tried to stay close to the game. I did television and radio color commentary for the XFL and for the Tampa Bay Buccaneers and Minnesota Vikings of the NFL. I love it so much I was even a volunteer football coach at Champlin Park High School in Minnesota for five years.

When you've been so close to the game for so long, you learn to love the positives of the game, but you also become intimately familiar with the negatives. The one negative that jumps off the screen every time I watch the game are the inevitable concussions. As a fan it is confusing to watch, because sometimes they are dealt with as a serious injury to the most important part of a person's anatomy—the brain—while other times they are joked about by the players, the announcers, the coaches, . . . nearly everybody. Which is it?

Christopher Nowinski's comprehensive, indisputable research has convinced me that these injuries are no joke. I met Chris when I was a visiting fellow at the Kennedy School of Government at Harvard University. (Yes, we are the only two Harvard-affiliated professional wrestlers in the world, but I'm the only one that taught there!) Chris "Harvard," as he is known, had a promising future with my former employer, Vince McMahon's World Wrestling Entertainment, before the concussions he sustained over the course of his athletic career turned his life upside down.

And while that may have been a loss for the wrestling world, it is unquestionably a gain for the sports community. He has turned his personal struggle into a quest to educate others on an injury that still seems to be as much of a mystery today as it was when I suffered my one serious concussion in a high school football game. I rammed heads with the fullback in the middle of the third quarter. The next thing I remembered was seeing the scoreboard—it said 5:51 was left in the *fourth* quarter. Apparently I had been pulled from the game and was sitting on the bench that whole time. As I became aware of my surroundings, everything I saw appeared to be at the end of a long tunnel. It was like having an out-of-body experience.

That day my coaches and trainer did the right thing by keeping me out of the game while I was concussed. What this book exposes, and what creates a real sense of urgency, is that my experience may not be the norm. Chris's research shows that most concussions are going undiagnosed, and most athletes aren't getting proper treatment. Multiple concussions, especially left untreated, can lead to serious long-term problems, including depression and dementia.

I understand that football is a tough sport, and that half the game is about playing through pain and battling through injuries. You don't graduate Navy SEAL training without knowing how to push yourself. But even I know that toughness has its limits, especially when we're talking about a game where 95% of the players have not reached the age of maturity.

This is the kind of book that everybody who is a part of this game—or any contact sport—needs to read. It has critical information for current players, former players, and future players. It has important guidelines for the parents who give permission to their children to put that helmet on and for the coaches and trainers who are the guardians of those kids on the playing field. It has fascinating stories for the NFL fans who want to know why their heroes keep retiring year after year from post-concussion syndrome.

Chances are that if you play football, nothing terrible will happen to you. But chances are you *will* suffer at least one concussion every season. And the difficult truth is that each concussion can have serious consequences on its own, but that successive concussions can have even greater consequences. It is the responsibility of players and parents to learn what those consequences are and what can be done to prevent them. No one should take the field without a clear understanding of the risks of the game, especially when just a little education can prevent so much suffering over the course of a lifetime.

JESSE VENTURA

former governor of Minnesota
and former NFL commentator

CHAPTER 1

Football's Concussion Crisis

Here's what terrifies me. Twelve-year-old Kyle Lippo, a seventh-grade football player from Round Lake, Illinois, during a game told his coach he had a headache and asked to sit the rest of the game out. Five minutes later, the coach asked Kyle if he wanted to go back in. Kyle said no, because his headache was getting worse. Then he started crying, saying, "It hurts really bad!"

Kyle was rushed to a local medical center, where he was loaded onto an emergency helicopter and taken to Advocate Lutheran General Hospital. There, on September 27, 2003, the Boy Scout, trombone player, and student council representative died from head trauma.[1] [2]

A few weeks later, Osten Gill, a 16-year-old high school sophomore from Rushford, New York, collapsed on the team bus as it was returning from a junior varsity football game. He had complained of dizziness and nausea after being hit during the game, and had vomited on the sidelines and on the bus. Osten died at a hospital several hours later.[3]

Then in November of 2003, 17-year-old safety Edward Gomez drilled a wide receiver coming across the middle on fourth down, forcing a dropped pass. Gomez popped up, was congratulated by his teammates, and headed to the sideline. Moments later he lost consciousness and collapsed. He died days later.[4]

Unlucky teenagers with isolated head injuries, you might say. After all, it is true that the number of deaths in youth football and youth sports in general caused by head injuries seems low, but I soon learned that death isn't the only worry associated with brain trauma. I played football for Harvard, and I recently attended a black-tie dinner celebrating the 100th anniversary of Harvard Stadium—the nation's oldest football stadium. Among the famous people at the event was former Chicago Bear great Dan Jiggetts, Harvard class of 1976. Every Chicago sports fan knows Dan from his playing days and broadcasting career, and, since he and I lived within a few miles of each other while I was growing up, he had taken an interest in my career. We chatted that night, and he asked how my wrestling career was going (it was 2003, and I was working for Vince McMahon and World Wrestling Entertainment—the WWE). When I told him that I had been sidelined with post-concussion syndrome, he became very serious. He told me, "You don't want to mess with that. The players of my generation are all worried about the links they've found with Alzheimer's disease." This was the first I'd heard of that supposed link. I lost my appetite.

The more I looked into my concussion problem, the more I realized that I had never heard of *any* of the true dangers posed by head injuries. Nor had the rest of the United States, it seemed. Why? Because the organization with the most money to study concussions and the biggest stage from which to spread the message at this point hasn't shown the ability to publicize the truth about these devastating injuries. To do so might hurt not only its game, but also the youth programs that feed its league and guarantee its loyal audience. Instead of promoting the proper information on safety, it uses its bully pulpit only to protect its business interests. The organization? The National Football League.

▼▼▼

Curiously, my study of head injuries in youth and professional sports didn't start while I was playing football for Harvard, but while I was working for the WWE. "Holy shit, kid! You okay?" was the first thing I heard after the kick to the head that led to the end of my wrestling career. The referee, Nick Patrick, leaned in, trying to figure out if I'd survived. Moments before, Bubba Ray Dudley's boot had met my chin with enough force to make the Hartford Civic Center explode. Or that's what it looked like to me as I lay on my back in the middle of the ring. Something was wrong with my vision. I didn't know where I was, what was happening around me, or why I was staring up at fuzzy-looking lights on the distant ceiling of a gigantic arena— I only knew that something was terribly wrong. I looked to the side, and saw thousands of people staring back at me. I gazed back up at Nick. I didn't want to move. My head felt like it was in a vice.

Then, a three-hundred-pound man with a crew cut and army fatigues appeared out of the fog—ready to squash me. I braced myself for the impact.

Crash! My head hurt more. Instead of rolling off of me, he hooked my leg, and the referee started counting.

"One! Two!"

Why is he counting? Oh yeah, I'm in a wrestling match. But wrestling is fake, right? I should be safe, because this stuff is scripted.

But I can't remember the script.

"Kick out, kid!" Nick whispered to me. I jerked the militant off me before the ref reached the count of three. I felt like a panicky little kid lost in a crowd. Slowly I started to remember what was happening. *I'm in a tag-team match against the Dudley Boyz, my partner Rodney Mack is in my corner with our manager Theodore Long . . .* But, before this crowd of thousands of pumped-up WWE fans, I still couldn't answer the most important question: What comes next? I know I have to do *something*, but what?

▼▼▼

I was able to finish the match against the Dudleys (I lost), and I stumbled backstage, lay down on the cold cement floor, and tried to compose myself. I was coherent and aware of my surroundings, but I couldn't get past an odd, throbbing headache. After a half-hour or so, as the headache faded, I became concerned about performing in the show the next night. The doctor the WWE had hired for the night said, "You *might* have a concussion. Let's see how you feel when you get to the arena tomorrow."

I arrived at the Pepsi Center in Albany, New York, at about 5 P.M. the next day. I felt strange, but I wasn't in "pain." Feeling strange didn't meet my criteria to take the night off, so I told the doctor I felt fine, and started to get ready for my "tables match" with the Dudley Boyz. If you've watched wrestling, you know that for this type of match to end, somebody has to go through a table. Guess who that was going to be? That's right, me.

I crept into the ring apprehensively. I opened up the match, locking up with Bubba Ray Dudley. He attacked me with a forearm to the back. I barely felt it—on my back. But for some reason, my head went fuzzy again, the blood pounding so fiercely that I thought my head would explode.

After a Dudley Death Drop (or "3D") sent me smashing through the table to the great joy of the crowd, I crawled backstage and found another place to lie down. The headache was much, much worse. This time I saw a different doctor. Again, I was told that I *might* have suffered a concussion the day before, which could explain the pain. The doctor said he couldn't be sure because he hadn't been there the night before. The pain went away after another hour or so, and I felt well enough to leave the building.

After the match, I headed to New York City. I was scheduled to wrestle on Monday Night RAW at Madison Square Garden the next night, in front of millions of people. I had no idea that it would be my last televised wrestling match ever. And not even a good one at that. I looked so sluggish when I arrived at the arena that two WWE agents, Fit Finlay and Dean Malenko, who were aware of my head problems, changed my match, over my objection, into something quick and simple—with no chance of head trauma. I survived the match without incident.

▼▼▼

As a former college football player and a guy who couldn't shake recurring post-concussion syndrome, I couldn't stop thinking about all those high school football players who had died in 2003 from brain injuries. I continued to scour newspapers and the Internet for similar stories, and over time I began to see a pattern.

Jacob Snakenberg was a freshman football player at Grandview High School in Denver. During a game, Jacob mysteriously collapsed after what appeared to be a routine tackle that did not involve contact to the head. He died two days later, and a neurosurgeon who operated on him said he died from a recent blow to the head. In the days following his death, his friends revealed that Jacob had been suffering from headaches during the previous week, following a big hit to his head in his last game. His father told the press he had specifically asked Jacob if his head hurt during that week, as he was concerned after watching Jacob take that blow, but Jacob had denied it.[5]

Jacob's story reminded me of something I hadn't thought about in ten years. During my sophomore year of high school, I played for a coach who had lost his own son to a head injury on the football field. I vaguely remember my former athletic trainer used to mention it every preseason. I called him to get more details. "Kurt Thyreen got a concussion in a game. He didn't tell anyone," Hersey High School trainer Hal Hilmer explained. "We later found out from his friends that his head hurt so much that week that he couldn't play his trumpet in band class. No one bothered to tell us or the coaches. He took the field for the next game, took a hit to the head that ruptured a blood vessel, and passed away."

There seemed to be something extremely dangerous about getting hit in the head again shortly after suffering a concussion. I read that 16-year-old Californian Michael Pennerman, a cousin of 1994 Heisman Trophy winner Rashaan Salaam, fell unconscious on the sideline after being tackled during a football game. He had walked off the field on his own, gone over to his coach, and told him, "It feels like somebody is pulling me to the ground." He then collapsed, and died the next day. There was suspicion that he may have suffered a concussion earlier in the game, both due to his behavior in his last minute of consciousness and because his stepfather said he was taking hits all game long.[6]

Adam Melka, a 15-year-old linebacker at Arrowhead High School in Wisconsin and the son of a former University of Wisconsin football player, became dizzy and started vomiting on the sideline after a hit to the head. He was rushed to the hospital and underwent emergency brain surgery. His coaches and teammates were puzzled because the last hit he took wasn't an especially violent one. When Adam's father Jim rushed back from a hunting trip, he asked to see the game tape. While he agreed that the final hit wasn't anything special, he noticed that Adam took an extraordinary hit earlier in the game that left him visibly shaken. "You could see him go onto his knees and bend backwards," Mr. Melka said.[7] Adam survived, but has a long recovery ahead of him.

These articles introduced to me a new term, *second impact syndrome* (SIS), which describes the severe brain injury that athletes can suffer after they are hit in the head again soon after suffering a concussion.

▼▼▼

The fact that I wasn't familiar with SIS concerned me. After my head injury in Hartford, I ignored my headache, and participated in four more matches over the next few weeks.

I began to wonder just how many kids were playing through headaches like mine, or Kurt Thyreen's, or Jacob Snakenberg's, so I went to the Harvard Medical School library and started exploring the stacks. I found a medical study that recorded the number of concussions that high school football players suffer. The author was appointed to the National Football League's committee on mild traumatic brain injury, so I assumed he was the best. He collected data from athletic trainers, and reported that approximately 4 percent of football players suffer one concussion in a given season.[8] After having played the game for eight years, and reading those articles about the SIS kids, I was under the impression that football players didn't always tell trainers when their heads hurt. "The real number is probably a little higher," I thought, as I continued researching.

I came upon another study that focused on how many football players get headaches in games.[9] Doctors found that 19 percent of players suffered a headache during or after their most recent game, and 90 percent suffered a headache during or after at least one game that season. If I compared these two studies directly, they told me that approximately 1 out of every 50 headaches was caused by a concussion, and the other 49 were caused by something else. While I knew that having a headache didn't necessarily mean a concussion had occurred, those numbers didn't add up. Yet without more information I still couldn't be sure exactly how many concussions kids on the football field were suffering.

Then I found the study that connected the dots.[10] A doctor named Wayne Langburt sent a survey to high school football players (not trainers) in Pennsylvania after the 1999 season. Langburt asked how often they had experienced concussion symptoms that season. He made the survey anonymous, because he knew that players would hesitate to admit how many concussions they'd had if they thought their answers could be traced back to them. He also removed the term *concussion* from the survey and relied on a generic definition instead. He knew that many high school kids misunderstand what a concussion is, falsely believing it requires loss of consciousness. The results were shocking. The share of players who claimed to have suffered a concussion the previous season was not 4 percent, or even 14 percent, but was 47 percent! And these players didn't suffer just one concussion. Those who received concussions claimed an average of 3.4 each season.

That's a lot of potential Kurt Thyreens and Jacob Snakenbergs.

▼▼▼

I tried to make a comeback a few weeks after my last concussion. I was scheduled to wrestle four matches over a long weekend. After the first match, my head felt considerably worse than it had just hours before. The deterioration of my health continued after the second match, so much so that by the time I woke up on the third day, something was so obviously wrong with me that the WWE refused to let me perform in the third show that afternoon. That night I met my girlfriend at the time, Jessie, at my hotel in Indianapolis and went to sleep.

At some point during the night I woke up and realized I wasn't in the bed anymore. As I became aware of my surroundings, I found myself face-down on the floor, surrounded by shards of glass. I looked to my right. The nightstand was broken, and its glass surface was shattered. The lamp and the alarm clock that had been on the nightstand were on the ground. Jessie was yelling my name. "Chris! Chris!" "What?" I answered. "Are you okay?" Feeling no pain, and having no idea of what she'd just witnessed, I yelled back, "Why?"

I'd been having a nightmare. My screaming had woken her up, and when she opened her eyes she saw me standing on the bed, clawing at the wall as if I were trying to climb it. I was sweating, and all my muscles were engaged. Jessie tried yelling my name to wake me up. Then she tried pulling me back down in the bed, but she wasn't strong enough. After a few seconds of standing there, I apparently yelled, "Oh no, Jessie!" jumped off the bed, and crashed headfirst into the wall as if I were trying to catch something. I bounced off the wall and into the nightstand. After about ten seconds on the ground, I woke up.

I personally don't remember any of this. I only remember dreaming that Jessie was falling, and that I had tried to "save" her. When she told me what she'd seen, I was officially freaked out. I turned on the TV and stared at it until sunrise.

▼▼▼

Don't get me wrong. I think the NFL is fully aware of the problem of head injuries in football. They have to be, because a degenerative brain disease caused by playing football has been identified as a contributing factor in the premature death of at least one of its greatest players. In 2002, NFL Hall of Fame center Mike Webster died from a heart attack at age 50. Playing for the Pittsburgh Steelers for sixteen years, the undersized Webster was known for his ferociousness on the field. Yet he struggled severely after his playing career ended. He was unemployed, debt ridden, occasionally homeless, and even charged with forging prescriptions for Ritalin. He was fired from his job as an assistant strength and conditioning coach for the Kansas City Chiefs because he couldn't fulfill the responsibilities of the job. In 1999, he was diagnosed as being "punch drunk." An autopsy confirmed that he had chronic traumatic encephalopathy, a neurodegenerative condition that was usually reserved for boxers.[11] [12] [13]

In response to research revealing links between head injuries and neurological problems such as Alzheimer's disease, depression, and cognitive impairment, the Center for the Study of Retired Athletes at the University of North Carolina has surveyed thousands of former NFL players on their experiences with concussions. When the data was processed, it was discovered that the players' risk of suffering from these neurological illnesses was proportionate to how many concussions they'd had. Players who had suffered three concussions in their *lifetime* had more than three times the rate of clinically diagnosed depression and five times the rate of mild cognitive impairment, also known as pre-Alzheimer's disease.[14][15] Twenty percent of the group with at least three concussions was depressed, and 17 percent had significant memory impairment. Overall, former NFL players had a 37 percent greater chance of developing Alzheimer's disease than an average person who didn't butt heads for a living.[16]

In 2005, Terry Long, Mike Webster's former offensive line mate with the Pittsburgh Steelers, died at age 45 from what was later determined to be suicide. He had drunk antifreeze. Toward the end of his life, Long exhibited some of the same symptoms as Webster had: erratic behavior, poor decision making, and depression. At the time of his death, he was under investigation for setting fire to his failing chicken-processing factory for the insurance money. The neuropathologist that performed his autopsy found structural brain damage similar to Mike Webster's. He believes Long's neurological deterioration was also football related.

▼▼▼

Former NFL players appear to be in bad shape. The list of players forced to retire from multiple concussions grows every year, and now includes Troy Aikman, Steve Young, Wayne Chrebet, Ted Johnson, Al Toon, Chris Miller, Stan Humphries, Bill Romanowski, Merril Hoge, Frank Wycheck, Bob Christian, Dustin Johnson, Ed McCaffrey, and others. Based on this new trend, I was curious if the NFL—the corporation—was doing anything about it. What I found was surprising.

I was excited to learn that in 1992, the NFL formed a subcommittee to study mild traumatic brain injury.

I was disappointed to learn that the subcommittee appointed Elliott Pellman, the New York Jets team doctor, as chairman. Pellman is not a neurologist, went to medical school in Mexico, and in 2005 was caught by the

New York Times inflating his qualifications on his curriculum vitae.[17] While working for Major League Baseball, he was raked across the coals in the Congressional steroid hearings for defending MLB's steroid policies. He proved to have little functional knowledge of the program, including the important fact that players could disappear for up to an hour after they were notified of their random test, which gave them plenty of time to cheat the test.

I was excited to discover that the NFL was spending $2 million to fund studies on concussions in the NFL.

I was disappointed to read the results of those studies. Released in a multipart series in the medical journal *Neurosurgery*, not only were they poorly designed, but the conclusions they drew from the data went against just about every study on sports concussions published in the last twenty years, and their conclusions were consistently criticized by the peer reviewers. (Peer reviewers are experts in the field who are asked to provide analysis and interpretation of published studies, and often serve as the last line of defense in exposing poor research that somehow makes its way into print.)

I was encouraged to learn that following Terry Long's death, the current Pittsburgh Steelers' neurosurgeon—who had treated Terry while he was a player—checked his medical records and stated that Terry had never suffered a concussion as a Steeler. Without evidence of football concussions, the neurosurgeon concluded that Long's brain damage was unlikely to have been caused by football.

I was disappointed to read that another doctor found a letter written by that same Steelers' neurosurgeon revealing that Long had suffered a concussion during a game against the Houston Oilers in 1987. The concussion made him "lightheaded, dizzy, confused, and walk with an unsteady gait," and the doctor had recommended that Long take some time off.[18] When confronted with that letter, the neurosurgeon claimed he must have "overlooked" it when searching through Long's file.

▼▼▼

It's been almost three years since my last concussion. I have not returned to the wrestling ring due to persistent post-concussion problems, including terrible migraines that last about a week each month. Knowing what I now know about concussions, I'm concerned for my future. Yet my only choice is to wait and see what happens. It's too late for me.

But it's not too late for millions of amateur football players. More than 9 out of 10 concussions aren't being diagnosed, mainly because players, trainers, and coaches don't know what a concussion really is, and don't realize the damage that's caused by continuing to play following a concussion. Awareness is so poor that more than half of athletes at the *college* level have no knowledge of the possible consequences following a head injury.[19] And rather than acknowledge that the problem of concussions in football is bigger than previously believed, the discussion is being hijacked by groups that appear to have an agenda other than making football safer for children. The NFL, for example, continues to produce flawed studies that do not adequately diagnose concussions nor trace their long-term effects.[20][21] How does that affect your child? Well, while you can be sure that the youth of America hears the positive message of football through the NFL's enormous youth football promotional arm, they may not hear about the risks. And we probably won't ever hear that part of the story from the NFL, because its goal is to build a long-term market for watching football, which includes, according to one NFL employee, getting a football in the hand of every American youth by his sixth birthday.[22]

What you will learn is that few people know the truth about head injuries in sports, and even fewer people are able to protect you or your children. I hope that the information presented here will spark changes to youth and professional sports, despite the resistance that I know will come. Some day I hope to have a son, and I bet he'll want to play football. Deep down, I'm sure I'll want him to play, so he can have the same fun I had and face the same challenges I faced. Yet knowing what I now know, I'm not sure if I will be able to give him my blessing. I think there are too many unanswered questions. But I have the luxury of having a theoretical kid. You have a real one who needs real answers to real questions.

We can start by trying to solve this problem: Most concussion treatment guidelines advocate that an athlete rest for the remainder of the season if he suffers three concussions during that season. According to some studies, over 25 percent of football players report suffering more than three concussions every season.[23][24] Therefore, if we start diagnosing concussions correctly, and treating them based on the best current guidelines, more than one-quarter of every team won't finish the season. What should we do?

I am curious to find out.

CHAPTER *2*

The Downward Spiral

Overall I had six concussions. Most were pretty minor, and I was never knocked unconscious. After the last one, I pretty much had to retire. For about seven or eight months, I was really in an awful state and had no desire to do anything. I couldn't balance a checkbook, I couldn't remember what I was doing from room to room, and it was several months before I could actually drive a car. I had to start all over, and it was a 13-month process of getting all my cognitive skills back. I even had to learn how to read again.

I still get a lot of headaches. If I wake up with a headache, that's the way it's going to be that day. Bright lights bother me, and they can trigger a headache. It's tough because I'm on camera in front of the lights so much for ESPN. I don't think I've ever really gotten back to where I once was. Pretty close. But it took a lot of work, a lot of effort.

Merril Hoge, age 41, nine-year NFL veteran

I could never voluntarily take myself out of a game. I know I should, and everyone tells me that if I am feeling bad to come out . . . but I keep going until the coach tells me to come off or I drop. If I felt pain in my knee or in my ankle, or got a "ding," I would keep playing with it until it became serious — until something really happened.

Steve, age 16, high school sophomore

I can relate to those kids who feel compelled to keep going after their first concussion. My own experience—before I was given a full diagnosis—was a blurry nightmare. Literally. My leap out of bed was only the first of many bizarre nighttime incidents, and when I couldn't follow conversations during the day, I knew I was in trouble. But I kept competing, so I can understand what motivates kids to go back in the game even when they're seeing stars or the sky has changed colors. In contact sports, both coaches and athletes ask one question: "Are you hurt, or are you injured?" Because if you're just hurt, you're supposed to get back in there.

In many ways, that's how I succeeded at Harvard, and that's how I intended to succeed in the WWE.

▼▼▼

My love affair with football began in 1992, at the tender age of 13. Growing up in the Chicago suburb of Arlington Heights, Illinois, I learned to live for Friday night games under the lights at John Hersey High School. As a 6'3", 160-pound beanpole, I somehow found success as a middle linebacker, and I captained my team as a 6'5", 230-pound senior defensive end.

I was lucky enough to be recruited by Harvard University, where I played for four more years, including the 1997 Ivy League Championship season. Harvard, like all the Ivy League schools, doesn't offer athletic scholarships, but the educational opportunity was too great to pass up. So were the dining halls: I benefited from Harvard's all-you-can-eat system and became a 295-pound defensive tackle, earning honorable mention All-Ivy League accolades as a junior and making second team All-Ivy as a senior. I also graduated *cum laude* with a degree in sociology.

When I was younger, I thought football was the greatest sport ever invented. It combines intelligence, power, grace, speed, collisions, and pure, unadulterated violence. Eleven dedicated men work together on the field, their success dictated by a willingness to sacrifice personal glory for the good of the team. The lessons that football teaches its players and the entertainment it gives its fans are unparalleled in American team sports. There's no doubt that it has surpassed baseball as America's true pastime. Football taught me what I believe to be the simplest and most important maxim for success: In football, and in life, you're guaranteed to get knocked down. What separates us is what happens next. Will you get back up and get in there?

▼▼▼

Shortly after I sustained my final concussion, we had a show in Poughkeepsie, New York. I was to team up with Rodney Mack. As I packed for the trip, I was weighed down by the knowledge that I wasn't physically prepared for the show, but it never seriously crossed my mind to not wrestle. This was my job, and the fans were expecting me. Besides, the WWE would have had to shuffle the card around me at the last minute, drawing attention to my asking for a night off for a headache and feeling sluggish. I tried to imagine how they would react to that request, considering the kinds of injuries other wrestlers have endured in order to perform.

- Stone Cold Steve Austin was dropped on his head in a 1997 match. He broke his neck, and was a transient quadriplegic for 90 seconds. He said, "By all rights, I should have just laid there and waited for the MDs to come and give me the proper assistance. But I was thinking of the business, I was thinking of the show. I was looking to finish the match. Finally I started getting some movement back. I couldn't crawl on my hands; I could barely crawl on my elbows . . . I rolled up Owen (for the pin to finish the match)." [1]

- Former Olympic Gold Medalist Kurt Angle chose to postpone surgery on his broken neck to wrestle at Wrestlemania XIX. The entire arena knew that if he got hit the wrong way, he could be paralyzed. Angle was also knocked unconscious once in a WWE Heavyweight Championship triple-threat match—where three wrestlers compete in the ring at once. He was carried backstage while the other two wrestlers improvised a new match. When he regained consciousness, he stumbled back down the ramp, got back in the ring, and, despite the fact that he didn't know where he was or what was going on, managed to finish the match with the help of the other wrestlers. He still doesn't remember doing it.

- Former WWE Champion Brock Lesnar, working with Kurt Angle at Wrestlemania XIX, was injured while attempting a "shooting-star press" off the top rope. "I was a good 10, 12 feet off the mat on my jump, and I landed smack on my forehead and face. I weigh 290 pounds, so you can just imagine the force and the momentum of that. When I hit, I don't remember anything because I got a concussion. I won the match, but I couldn't tell you what happened." [2] He was back wrestling within two weeks.

- Former WWE Champion Triple H tore his quadriceps muscle in the middle of a match. Even so, he continued to wrestle for another five minutes because he wanted to finish the match in a way that was best for the storyline.

As these heroic performances ran through my mind, I decided there was no way I could ask for the night off. But when I arrived at the arena, I found I didn't have a choice. Apparently, I looked like such a mess that the trainer and doctor refused to let me wrestle. They were onto something. The next day I had to carry my bags up a flight of stairs to get into the arena in Syracuse, and I had to stop every few steps to keep from passing out. I took that night off, too. Sunday I sat out in Elmira, and at RAW in Buffalo on Monday I finally got some serious medical attention.

I was experiencing a lot of pain in the back left side of my head, and the doctors were worried that I may have suffered a subdural hematoma, meaning that my brain was bleeding inside my skull, which can be fatal. That afternoon I was sent to get a CT scan on my brain, and it showed no bleeding. I was immediately seen by a neurosurgeon, who told me that I had *probably* suffered a minor concussion the previous week. He asked me if I'd ever had a concussion before. I told him no. Based on the assumption that this was my first concussion, he recommended that I take a few days off, and predicted that I would be fine in a week or two. My frustration at having to wait was growing. This was *not* how I had gotten my job, *not* how I had made it this far, and if this continued, I was certain my dreams would end.

▼▼▼

Wrestling for the WWE wasn't exactly my dream growing up, mainly because of my mother. She didn't allow me to watch wrestling because she thought that just watching it would cause brain damage. Oh, the irony. I became hooked on wrestling the summer before my senior year of college, while living on-campus to train for the upcoming football season. I had five roommates. We each weighed over 250 pounds, and were crammed into a two-bedroom place with one television. Since the other guys never miss wrestling, I was forced to watch it Monday and Thursday nights. At first I resisted, but I slowly fell in love with the show, tuning in to watch The Rock, Stone Cold Steve Austin, and Kurt Angle battle for supremacy.

Coming out of college, I wasn't one of the lucky few hundred football players who make the pros, so I was forced to give up the game. My first real job after college was a summer internship with the consulting firm Trinity Partners, LLC. I worked for a Harvard football alum, and focused on commercialization strategy in the pharmaceutical and biotech industries. Most of the firm's employees were Ivy League graduates with science and economics degrees, so I was an anomaly with my sociology background. But I guess I learned enough in college and on the job to keep up—I still work there.

Strangely enough, the owner of Trinity Partners, John Corcoran, was a huge wrestling fan, and used to consult for Vern Gagne and the American Wrestling Association (AWA). We started to talk wrestling in the office. One day, as John and I were debating the merits of the Stone Cold Stunner vs. The People's Elbow as finishing maneuvers, he asked me if I'd ever considered becoming a professional wrestler. I hadn't. Since I'd dabbled in theater, and had had success in athletics, John thought I could make it.

I said, "I don't know. I have a good job here."

He said, "Work here parttime and go to wrestling school fulltime. Give it a shot and we'll see what happens."

With that kind of golden parachute, how could I say no?

I enrolled at Killer Kowalski's Wrestling Institute in November of 2000. I loved it—each practice was more fun than the one before. Three months into my training, MTV and World Wrestling Entertainment announced a new reality television show called *Tough Enough*. The show set out to find and train future superstars for the WWE while giving the world a glimpse of what it takes to become a professional wrestler. The show combined elements of *The Real World* and *Survivor*. Thirteen contestants (eight males and five females) would live in a house together, and their lives and WWE training would be taped. One person would be eliminated every week. I joined the cast.

The thirteen of us were put through grueling six-hour training sessions every day. The toughness and confidence I had learned playing football at Harvard got me through to the end. The trainers discovered that while most of the cast members were crumbling both physically and emotionally, they couldn't break me. I knew how to work through pain and adversity—how to play hurt. For example, after the show I found out I had torn a ligament in my wrist in the first week of training. It had hurt the entire time, but I knew I couldn't stay in the contest with a cast, so I just taped it and didn't tell anyone about it. Unfortunately, toughness did not equal talent, and when two contestants were awarded contracts with World Wrestling Entertainment at the end of the show, I wasn't one of them.

Still, I wasn't dissuaded. Even if the WWE didn't know it yet, I knew I could become good enough to make it in that business. Six months later my perseverance paid off and the WWE hired me. In 2002, I made my debut in front of five million viewers on Monday Night RAW as Chris "Harvard" Nowinski, the Ivy League snob. I became known for taunting the audience for its lack of intelligence. Sometimes I would recite poetry from the ring. My favorite poem may be one I recited in Moncton, New Brunswick, Canada. (To understand the rhyming scheme, you need to know that Canadians say "grade 3" instead of "third grade.")

> Roses are red,
> Violets are blue,
> The reason I'm talking so slowly,
> Is because no one in Moncton has passed grade 2

I'd often apply my education during a match. In a Hardcore match in Bridgeport, Connecticut, I assaulted Al Snow with a human skeleton, ripped off the skull, got down on bended knee, and began reciting *Hamlet.* Those were good times.

▼▼▼

I was so frustrated by the runaround I felt I was getting from doctors over the nine days since Bubba's boot that I was ready to blow off the Buffalo neurosurgeon. But I didn't. When I returned to the arena after my CT scan, Vince McMahon, the chairman and the heart and soul of the WWE, made the executive decision that, although my diagnosis still wasn't clear, I wouldn't be allowed to wrestle that night or get hit at ringside. I was willing to wrestle, and I am now thankful that he took my long-term future into consideration even when I didn't. That night I accompanied my tag-team partner at ringside for his singles match, and the increase in my blood pressure just from cheering him on nearly knocked me out. I had a throbbing headache when I got backstage.

I went to see a neurologist when I got back home to Boston. He advised me to take a week or two off, and also recommended that I not get back into the ring until I was asymptomatic while at full exertion for a few days (meaning that I felt normal when I was working out). After about ten days, I still wasn't feeling better, but I was getting restless. Since all the doctors had told me that I should have been feeling better by now, I began to doubt myself—I wondered if maybe the symptoms were all in my head. So with my mind playing tricks on me, and a conscious fear of losing my position in the company, I lied to the doctor and got myself medically cleared. I boarded a plane for our show that weekend in Omaha, Nebraska.

My partner, Rodney Mack, and I were scheduled for a tag match against Rosey and Tommy Dreamer. As we prepared for the match, I knew that something was wrong. I was having trouble remembering the few prepared sequences of moves that we'd talked over; this had never happened to me before. One of the few things I had going for me in the ring was my memory—I never made mistakes. I was worried about performing our match. I didn't want to embarrass myself in front of my coworkers or the crowd, and I didn't want to make a mistake in the ring that would injure my opponents or me. There is truly very little margin for error in this business.

Fear of embarrassment from backing out just before the match overwhelmed my thoughts of self-preservation.

I told myself, "You felt this way as you got on the plane, rented a car, and drove to the arena. The match is only an hour away. Sorry, pal, but it's way too late to change your mind."

I did the only thing I felt I could do to help myself: I asked the other guys if I could "take it easy" that night, and not take many bumps. As a rookie, I was taking my life in my own hands—the other three guys were older veterans, and would have been justified in ignoring my plea. From the looks on their faces, I thought they were going to beat me up right then and there. But because they were good guys, they didn't, and I survived the match.

The next morning we flew to Green Bay.

Tommy asked, "Do we need to take it easy on you again?"

"Yes, please, sir," I answered, to a pair of rolling eyes. We worked a similar match that night, and again I walked away in a slight daze with only a headache.

But something changed overnight. The next morning I woke up feeling miserable. I met the rest of the wrestlers at the airport and hopped on a plane to Indianapolis, Indiana, where we were to rent cars to drive to a Sunday afternoon show in Terre Haute. By the time we landed in Indianapolis, I was having trouble focusing.

At the baggage claim, my tag team's manager, Theodore Long, pleaded with me in his best fatherly voice, "You don't look so hot. Your head's messed up. You shouldn't wrestle."

I was finally starting to agree. I drove to the arena with our head of security, Jimmie Tilles, but didn't talk for most of the ride because I just couldn't keep up with the conversation. By the time we arrived at the arena, Theodore and Rodney had already warned the head road agent, Black Jack Lanza, that something was wrong with me. He saw me in the parking lot and told me that I wasn't wrestling that night. When Jimmie heard that, he exclaimed, "Thank goodness." Part of me was relieved, and part of me was concerned that this would set my career back.

I went back to the hotel, and that's the night I jumped off the bed. My girlfriend Jessie escorted me to the arena the next morning. I was met at the door, and told that I wasn't getting in the ring again until they knew what was wrong with me. I was no longer in any mood to argue. Vince McMahon was kind enough to pull me aside and tell me to take as much time as I needed to heal.

He said, "It's not worth it. You only have one brain."

I ran into head agent John Laurinaitis, who scolded, "Ya gotta tell us when you're hurt."

As I continued the long walk to the locker room, I passed Stephanie McMahon, the "Billion Dollar Princess." She's Vince's daughter and head of the creative department. She repeated Vince's offer to take as much time as I needed. During the conversation, Jessie told Stephanie about the incident at the hotel the night before. Stephanie's jaw dropped. I was uncomfortable, so I tried to lighten the mood by pointing out how romantic it was that I yelled Jessie's name when I jumped, and that I was trying to save her from falling in my dream. Neither woman was impressed.

There was a physician at the show, and he told me that sleep disturbance could be a side effect of a concussion. He asked me if I had a history of concussions.

I said, "I've been dinged here and there, but nothing I would call a concussion."

"Well, without a previous history of concussion problems, you should probably be fine in a week or two."

He handed me a prescription for muscle relaxers. "This should make you sleep more soundly. We don't want you to hurt yourself."

I flew home the next morning, expecting to be out for a couple of weeks and to return to the ring without missing a beat. Since nobody had told me not to work out, I started going back to the gym. About twenty minutes into each workout, my head would pound like never before. Being bull-headed, I tried to ignore it. But after a few days the feeling became overwhelming.

It was the strangest sensation. I could be in the middle of a set of bench presses, and after a few repetitions I would feel so odd, both physically and emotionally, that I would lose my desire to lift the weights off my chest. My trainer, Walter Norton Jr., would have to rack the weight for me. It wasn't pain, it was more like intense apathy. At that moment, I wouldn't have cared if somebody had dropped a weight on my face. I began to fear that feeling, and I stopped working out.

The neurologist I was seeing at the time kept recommending longer and longer periods of rest. We chose to not medicate my headaches with Tylenol, ibuprofen, or prescription drugs because the doctor was concerned that it would mask the pain and I would begin exercising again too quickly.

The stress of not knowing what was wrong with me or how to cure my heachaches was devastating, and I became depressed. Concentrating, reading, and carrying on a conversation made my head hurt. I couldn't even pass the time and lift my spirits by hanging out with friends or watching a funny movie because laughing gave me a splitting headache. That was the worst. Laughter is the best medicine, my ass.

On top of the emotional problems, my memory was off. I couldn't remember people's names, socially or professionally. A few months after the injury I was backstage at a WWE show in Chicago with the Brooklyn Brawler, Steve Lombardi. He was giving me a good-natured ribbing me about my concussion, and as a joke he started pointing to people and asking, "Remember his name? Remember her name?" It was funny because the people he pointed to were some of the most recognizable wrestlers in the world—like Triple H and Ric Flair—people I'd worked with for a couple of years and had idolized for even longer. It stopped being funny when I struggled to come up with their names. At one point I paused so long that he stopped walking and said, "You're kidding with me, right?"

I put on my biggest grin.

"Of course, Brawler."

I wasn't kidding. I was in big trouble.

▼▼▼

It was clear I wasn't getting better, and I was reaching the end of my rope. Some days I wouldn't get off the couch. Some days I would try to go to bed at 5 P.M. because my head hurt and I had nothing to distract me from the pain. But then I would dread waking up 4 A.M.—alone, in the dark, and with the headache. My girlfriend traveled three nights a week for work and wasn't always around, so I mostly suffered alone. My friends tried to be there for me, but after a while their patience for my constant misery grew thin. Football season was starting. At least I could watch that.

But by wintertime, with all that I would learn about concussions that season, I couldn't watch football in the same way. The joy of the big hit was gone for me.

CHAPTER *3*

My Concussion Education

One of the really frightening things was the night following the 1994 NFC champi-onship game between San Francisco and Dallas. Troy Aikman played for Dallas; they beat San Francisco and Aikman got a concussion. I visited him in the hospital room, and he asked me if he'd played in the game. I told him he did. He asked me how he had played. I said, "Well." He then wanted to know if winning that game meant that they were going to the Super Bowl. "Yes," I said. He asked when the Super Bowl would be played and where—I answered him, and he got really excited. His face brightened, and it was great.

Five minutes later, he asked me whether he'd played in the game that day, and if they'd won, and how he'd played, and whether that meant they were in the Super Bowl. I answered. Another ten minutes passed, and he asked me the same questions again. I thought for a while he was joking—but he wasn't. This went on, so I finally wrote down the most commonly asked championship game night questions.

Leigh Steinberg, Troy Aikman's agent

I have no recollection of any of this, but apparently after my concussion, while I was at the hospital, I asked my Mom for a lighter. I was a little warm and I wanted to set the sprinkler system off (to cool off). That's a little crazy, but the kicker is that my mom doesn't smoke and has never carried a lighter.

Nick Fisher, 17, high-school senior

I always related concussions to boxing. When I played, I didn't know they even ex-isted in the NFL. If they would have sat me in a room and said, "You cannot leave here until you guess the one mystery injury that could end your career," I'd still be in that room. I would never have thought concussions were part of football.

Merril Hoge, 41, nine-year NFL veteran

Part of my frustration was caused by a sense of vagueness—not just the cloudiness in my mind, but the kinds of answers I was getting from medical authorities. It seemed that there were few ways to accurately diagnose and describe what had happened to me, predict how long symptoms would persist, and chart a recovery course and time frame. That left me to wonder if my symptoms were all in my head. This made the calls from the WWE ever more difficult.

The WWE liaison would call every few days. The conversations grew short and routine:

"How are you feeling?"

"Terrible."

"All right, I'll check back in a few days."

They decided to send me to the "NFL and NHL experts." I flew to the Midwest and met with a bearded gentleman in his forties. We talked about how the injury happened, and then he gave me a laptop so I could take a new kind of concussion test—a computerized neurological assessment. Considered superior to a noncomputerized test because of its sensitivity to small changes, the program would ask a series of questions that measured things such as memory and reaction time.

In one section, I was asked to remember some black and white pictures and graphics. Later I was shown a larger group of pictures that included some from that earlier group. As pictures flashed on the screen, I was asked to press "yes" if I recognized a picture from the earlier group, and "no" if it was a new picture. About ten questions in, I started to sweat. At first, I answered "no" to each question because I didn't remember seeing the designs. After a while, it dawned on me that there was no way they could show me ten new images in a row, so there had to be some "yes" answers sprinkled in there somewhere—but I couldn't remember having seen a single one of the pictures. So I began randomly guessing.

The only reason I answered more than 50 percent of the questions correctly was that some images were repeated, and the program gave immediate "correct" or "incorrect" feedback. So while I couldn't remember if I'd already seen the image from the first pass through, I could remember if I'd answered the question correctly the first time.

When the doctor scored the test, he didn't seem worried. I'd scored very well on most sections, and he said that on one particular section I'd scored in the same range as "your average NFL player." I told him, point blank, that I had guessed on those answers. He shrugged it off. He said that without a baseline test score (my score if I'd taken the test before the concussion), there was no way to be sure if my score was lower now than it would have been then. Since I was within normal ranges, I think he thought that I was a worrywart.

As we wrapped up the consultation, I heard again that there was no reason to believe that I wouldn't be better in a couple of weeks.

I left the office frustrated. Another doctor, another vague answer. I was starting to think that this whole concussion treatment concept was suspect. In football, when I had broken a bone or tore a ligament, a doctor would touch something and ask, "Does this hurt?" I would say yes or no. Then he'd do something else, and ask, "How about this?" Eventually he'd figure out what was wrong, take an x-ray or MRI, and tell me, "If you can take the pain, you can play" or "The bone will heal sufficiently for you to play in three to four weeks."

But a doctor couldn't just touch my head now to identify the source of the pain. I was told that MRI's and CT scans were not sensitive enough to detect concussions. And the computerized neuropsychology tests were relatively useless without a baseline score. When a doctor would perform a clinical exam, he'd ask, "Was there a loss of consciousness?" I'd answer "No." Invariably, the doctor would say, "Hmmm," and scratch his chin. He'd ask me to stand up, and then he'd put me through a physical routine much like a drunk-driver test from the television show *Cops*. The doctor would take out the old-school reflex hammer and hit me a few times. I'd flinch. He'd ask me questions to test my mental dexterity. Over time I learned to count backward by 7 from 100. Sometimes I'd get asked about the symptoms that I was experiencing. That was especially frustrating, because I didn't know what symptoms were relevant. How could I possibly know what to say?

As the doctors were running out of tests, I was running out of hope. I'd wandered into a medical "no-man's land." I looked normal from the outside and could carry on a conversation, so these experts seemed to assume that I was fine. I was the only one who believed that something was wrong.

All I knew was that I had a headache, bright lights bothered me, I hadn't had a good night's sleep in weeks, I could barely remember my appointment dates, I was depressed, and I wasn't getting better. And to top it all off, I didn't know how, or if, I'd ever recover.

▼▼▼

My luck was about to change. Through a friend, I learned that one of the world's leading concussion experts worked at a hospital just a half-hour from my home. I figured he was my last hope, so I made up my mind not to leave his office until I had some answers.

Dr. Robert Cantu had an impressive résumé. When I saw him, he was chief of neurosurgery at Emerson Hospital in Concord, Massachusetts, co-director of the Neurological Sports Injury Center at Brigham and Women's Hospital in Boston, Massachusetts, the medical director for the National Center for Catastrophic Sports Injury Research, vice-president of the National Operating Committee on Standards for Athletic Equipment (NOCSAE), the NOCSAE liaison to the NFL Commissioner's Mild Traumatic Brain Injury (mTBI) committee, and a former president of the American College of Sports Medicine. He sat on the editorial board of multiple medical journals, and he had authored over three hundred scientific publications and nineteen books on neurology and sports medicine. He also had the prestigious honor of being the first person to publish return-to-play guidelines for sports concussions (in 1986).

But if I'd learned anything during my ordeal, it was that a good résumé was no guarantee of good doctoring. So when I arrived at his office, I began looking for clues as to whether this guy was legit. From the looks of his waiting room, it was difficult to tell whether he was any better than the others I'd seen. There were autographed pictures of famous athletes on the wall, but I'd been to offices with more. I saw the books on his shelves that he'd written, but I had no idea how good they were.

To begin the consultation, Dr. Cantu gave me a piece of paper with a list of symptoms on it. He asked me to mark on a scale of one to five those symptoms that were bothering me at that moment. The sheer number and range of symptoms was surprising. There were twenty or so symptoms on the list, everything from nausea to irritability. During the eleven years that I'd played football and wrestled, I thought that to have a concussion, you had to be knocked unconscious or senseless. Apparently I'd been misinformed. A commonly accepted definition of concussion is a "trauma-induced alteration in mental status that may or may not involve a loss of consciousness."[1] The NFL uses the following definition.

> A traumatically induced alteration in brain function manifested
> by an alteration of awareness or consciousness, including but not
> limited to a loss of consciousness, "ding," sensation of being
> dazed or stunned, sensation of "wooziness" or "fogginess,"
> seizure, or amnesic period, and by symptoms commonly associ-
> ated with postconcussion syndrome, including persistent
> headaches, vertigo [dizziness], light-headedness, loss of balance,

unsteadiness, syncope [LOC], near-syncope, cognitive dysfunction, memory disturbances, hearing loss, tinnitus [ringing in the
ears], blurred vision, diplopia [double vision], visual loss, personality change, drowsiness, lethargy, fatigue, and inability to perform usual daily activities.[2]

Dr. Cantu told me I got a score of 15 on the symptom test. That meant
I wasn't doing horribly, but I wasn't exactly a model of health, either. I worried that he would tell me, "You're cleared to wrestle when you're a 5 on
this test," and then it would be up to me to determine when I was a 5, and
then I would lie to myself about how poorly I felt so I could go back to
work. So I launched a preemptive strike.

I asked Dr. Cantu, "Why do I have a score of 15? What's going on in
my head?"

During this meeting and the weeks that followed, Dr. Cantu would
blow my mind (no pun intended) about concussions. To answer my questions, he started with the basics: A concussion is actually not defined by a
physical injury, but by a loss of brain *function* that is induced by trauma.[3]
Thinking of the concussion as a brain malfunction or as an alteration
in mental status—and not as a mysterious injury inside my head that
couldn't be detected by conventional tests—was much easier for me to
comprehend.

I immediately thought of a couple of wrestlers I'd worked with. At age
18, Renee Dupree was the youngest wrestler ever signed by the WWE. We
came up through the organization's developmental system at the same
time, and became friends. Once we were working a show somewhere in
America's heartland (with or without concussions it's hard to keep track of
all the places we've been) and word got backstage that Renee was hurt.
Security and the trainer helped him out of the ring, and I walked with him
to the locker room. He was bleeding above his eye, and totally out of it.
The trainer went to get supplies to clean up the cut, and asked me to stay
with Renee. Since injuries are so common in wrestling, no one was paying
much attention to us. Renee looked up, noticed me there, and asked, "Did
I wrestle yet?"

"Yes," I answered.

"How was the match? Was it good?"

I told him. "Yes, very good."

"Good, good," he said. For about thirty seconds he stared straight ahead. Then he asked me, "Did I wrestle yet?"

"Uh, yes."

"How was the match? Was it good?"

I told him. "Yep, very good."

"Good," he said again. Thirty seconds later, he asked again. The trainer came back by the fourth go-round. An hour later Renee seemed relatively normal, and the next day he apologized profusely for "whatever he might have said after the match."

Bubba Ray Dudley had a similar but more tragic story. He suffered a concussion during a match just months after his mother had died. Her death had hit him hard, but he had kept his emotions bottled up to stay strong for the rest of his family. When he got backstage after suffering the concussion, his malfunctioning brain was suddenly focused on his mother, but he could only remember that she had been sick, not that she had passed away. He asked Tommy Dreamer and Spike Dudley, "How's my mother?" Although they didn't understand why he was asking the question, they dutifully answered, "She passed away a few months ago." For the first time since is mother died, Bubba Ray began to cry. Then, oddly, he stopped crying and started talking about something else. A few minutes later, he asked another wrestler, "How's my mother?" "She passed away a few months ago," he was told. He began crying again, as if hearing the news for the first time. He stayed in a hotel that night with Dreamer, who was asked to keep an eye on him. Dreamer told me this cycle repeated over thirty times with various people over the course of the evening. Each person thought they were doing the right thing by answering the question honestly. When Tommy finally had Bubba away from everyone, he decided it was too painful to let continue. When Bubba Ray would ask again, Tommy would answer "She's fine." Bubba doesn't remember any of it.

I asked Dr. Cantu what causes this "malfunction."

He said, "To begin, you have to picture the concussion not just as an *event*, but also as a *process*."[4]

He then went on to explain the difference. Physical damage to the brain structure is an example of an *event*. This *may* occur at the time of injury, and is usually restricted to more severe concussions.[5] The physical injury is caused by two mechanisms. First, the brain can smash against the inside of the skull. In this case, the damage to the brain is complicated by the fact that the inside of the skull isn't smooth, but has ridges of bone. Second, the wave of energy that passes through the brain tissue can crush, stretch, and shear brain cells and the nerve fibers connecting them (which are called axons).[6]

An example of the *process* is sometimes called the "neurometabolic cascade of concussion."[7] If the impact is strong enough to trigger a concussion, the brain immediately begins going through chemical and metabolic changes.[8][9][10][11][12] It's a complicated process. I asked David Hovda, PhD, the director of the UCLA Brain Injury Research Center, and internationally known for his work on traumatic brain injuries, to explain. He told me, "When the brain gets pushed or pulled or moved violently, all the cells in the brain fire. It's kind of like a small seizure. When that happens, chemicals, called neurotransmitters, are released. These are the chemicals we use in the brain to communicate from one cell to another. When they communicate all at once, they activate receptors, and these receptors spill out ions, which is normally what they do—but not to this degree."

Dr. Hovda explained that the concussion causes potassium ions to rush out of the cells and flood the brain, while calcium ions rush inside the cells. "The cells activate pumps to send one ion—potassium—back in, and another ion—calcium—back out," he continued. "This requires energy, and that energy is derived from metabolism, or from utilizing the fuel in the brain. The brain fuel used originally is glucose, so the brain will burn a lot of glucose to get its ions back where they belong." But the calcium impairs the cells, and the brain can't create the energy needed to fire the pumps. Dr. Hovda explained, "When calcium comes in, it messes up the machinery that the cell has to make the energy to drive the pumps. So after a concussion, you have an increased need for energy, but you have a deficiency in the ability to make energy."

Essentially, the brain is now running on low batteries, so it doesn't function as well. "The cells turn off and become quiet," he told me. "When you do a metabolic study, the brain has essentially shut down, so the individual will exhibit symptoms as if the brain is not working well. He has a hard time remembering or learning new things, and he'll feel tired and lethargic for a long period of time." All this action occurring in the brain then manifests itself as a wide range of acute symptoms for the concussed athlete.

Symptom	% Reporting at Time of Injury
Headache	92%
Dizziness	72%
Blurred vision	67%
Disorientation	58%
Confusion	56%
Disequilibrium	44%
Nausea/vomiting	39%
Anterograde amnesia	31%
Neck pain	31%
Photophobia	31%
Sleepiness	28%
Fatigue	25%
Loss of consciousness	19%
Retrograde amnesia	19%
Irritability	17%

Source: Guskiewicz KM, Ross SE, Marshall SW. Postural Stability and Neuropsychological Deficits After Concussion in Collegiate Athletes. *Journal of Athletic Training* 36:3 (2001): 263–373.

The symptoms themselves will carry on for varying periods of time, depending on a person's individual brain chemistry, the severity of the injury, prior concussions, the number and severity of secondary collisions after the first concussion, and other factors. People like Nick Fisher know this all too well.

When I was introduced to Nick, he was a 17-year-old senior at Abington High School, in Abington, Massachusetts. A three-sport athlete and member of the National Honor Society, Nick was primed to be a starting wide receiver in his senior season. But a concussion in practice changed everything. I spoke with him four months after his injury. Since we seemed to be going through the exact same thing, we formed an immediate bond.

Nick was feeling miserable the day we met and wasn't trying to hide it. "Senior year was supposed to be my time to shine. I'd paid my dues. The day I got hurt, we were doing special teams in practice. I don't remember this, but apparently a kid came down, then popped me right up underneath my chin, knocking me out cold. I remember the ambulance a little bit because it was scary. I was strapped down, I couldn't move, I was all by myself.

No one went with me to the hospital. That was just terrifying. The only other thing I remember about getting hurt is that the sky was green and the ground was blue. That's about it.

"The coach seemed kind of happy. He said, 'I like calling the ambulance at least once or twice a season.' Thanks, coach." Nick shook his head in disgust. "I've known him since I was born, and I still have a lot of respect for him and consider him a friend. But he's old school. 'Play through it.' For a whole week I was groggy, out of it, tired. From September until November I pretty much had a headache that never went away—until I started taking pills. They put me on the type of stimulant used to treat ADHD so I can maintain my focus at school.

"I kept going to school, but I wasn't very effective there. I was in "la-la" land, and I just couldn't follow the logic. I'd get a few steps in and ask myself, 'What am I doing?' I started losing focus and my grades slipped. The pills seemed to help, but I couldn't sleep while I was taking them. I worked on three hours of sleep for months. Since I never felt tired, I didn't think there was anything wrong with that."

Nick had serious concerns for his future. "I want to go to Northeastern University, major in criminal justice, and become a state trooper," he told me. "When I applied, my doctor had to write a letter explaining the drop in my grades. He explained that I hadn't gotten treatment, but now with treatment the situation was being resolved, and I would hopefully be able to regain what I'd lost. Hopefully. I felt bad asking him to write me a letter, because it felt like a crutch. A doctor has to help me get into college? That doesn't seem right. I want to earn my own way.

"I worry that if I become a policeman or if I go into the Army, I might see something and react completely differently than someone who hasn't gotten his head whacked a couple times. Maybe the chemical balance in my brain has been thrown off. If I see a guy with a gun, or if I see some guy beating his wife, am I just going to snap, and start shooting at him or something? I think that after enough blows to the head, you turn into a different person. You don't register things in the same way, or have the same thoughts or reactions. I don't want anyone to think that I'm bonkers right now, but it's something I worry about.

"I don't want to burden anybody with my concussion, so I don't tell anyone what I'm feeling. I put on a façade. I try to act like I was before the injury, but I'm definitely a changed person. I have a lot less enthusiasm about stuff. The kids at school say things. It's *the* joke. Everybody: teachers, coaches. . . . Kids might be goofing off at lunch and this one teacher will say, 'Stop throwing stuff. You might hit Fish and he might hurt himself.' I kind of understand where they're coming from, because they don't know. There's nothing out there that would help them understand a concussion."

Nick was sending me on an emotional roller coaster. He went on. "I'm not the person I used to be. Without sports, what do I have to work for? How do I talk about this, about everything that I feel? I live my life for 17½ years one way, and then, bam! September 8, here I am. I'm completely depressed. 'Is there anything wrong?' they ask. 'No, I'll be all right, it's just one of those days.' I've just been having one of those days for two months. I'm not bitter at the game, I'm bitter at the circumstances. I would have liked to play this year."

Thanks to Dr. Cantu, I began to understand what had happened to me and why I was feeling as I did. But like Nick, I was plagued with symptoms and with questions: How long would my symptoms last? What would the long-term effects be? Would I ever be normal again? Would I be able to get back in the ring?

CHAPTER *4*

The Road to Recovery

I got a concussion, took a few days off, and returned to play before I had completely re-covered. I took another hit a couple of weeks later, and I took what I call a standing eight count. There wasn't any great magnitude, with no amnesia or loss of conscious-ness. I never reported that only for the fact that I didn't know to report anything.

Three weeks later, I got the same type of collision. That one was very similar—I didn't lose consciousness but I don't remember anything. I went back to the huddle for a few plays and then came to the sideline.

My facemask had been bent across my face and cut my chin open. They put a crowbar in there to pull my facemask out so they could get my helmet off. They were just going to stitch my chin up and give me a new facemask. Even at that point they didn't know that I "wasn't there." They knew I was bleeding so they stitched me up, but when they were stitching me up, then they realized something was wrong.

We went to the locker room, and I stopped breathing. I stopped breathing for about fifteen seconds. I lost all my vital signs. They took me to intensive care. I stayed there for two days. I basically had to retire after that.

Merril Hoge, 41, nine-year NFL veteran

It became clear that there was such a thing as a "second concussion syndrome"—if a player got a concussion in game A, he was much more susceptible to a concussion if he got hit again in the head soon after. One week Steve Young got a concussion. The doctors asked him if he'd gotten a concussion, and he said, "No." They okayed him to play in the next game, and he got a second concussion. Getting two concussions was exponentially worse than getting one, and was enough to knock him out of the game.

Leigh Steinberg, Steve Young's agent

We're too focused on the "event." In a heart attack, there is an event; in a hip frac-ture, the broken bone is the event. With brain injury, after the initial impact, the damage is not done—after the initial injury, it can continue. That's what's so chal-lenging about these injuries.

Dr. Heechin Chae, MD

By now, I had a pretty clear understanding of what had happened inside my head right after the injury in Hartford. But to be honest, I was more concerned with *when* I would get better than *how*. Deep down, I knew that once I got better, I wouldn't care *how* it had happened. But no matter how much I wanted to feel better and move on with my life, I was stuck in a rut and I didn't know why. I thought that *when* I would recover was a function of the number of concussions I'd had. But for some reason that system wasn't working for me.

Therefore, I continued to take the offensive in my meeting with Dr. Cantu. As we discussed my medical history, he asked the obligatory, "How many concussions have you had?" I told him I'd had zero or one, mostly to see whether he had a different answer for each number. But instead of giving me a prognosis, he paused thoughtfully and asked another question.

"Well, how many times after a hit have you experienced any of the symptoms we just talked about?"

A light went on in my head. Due to my inability to think clearly, I hadn't connected how the new definition of concussion I'd just learned applied to my past. I could feel my brain reorganizing; hits that had previously been filed in my memory in a large folder labeled "getting my bell rung" were now being transferred to a much thinner "concussion" folder.

"In April, I was kicked in the head and blacked out for five or six seconds. Could that have been a concussion?" I asked.

"Describe what happened," he answered.

I began to tell the story. Two months prior to my last concussion, I was working a match in Louisville, Kentucky, when Nova (known today as Simon Dean), threw me into the ropes. I recall running toward the ropes, hitting a wrinkle in time, and then realizing that I was on my back in the middle of the ring. Nova picked me up by my hair, and I struggled to remember what I was supposed to do next. As we continued, I had to ask him, over and over, "What's next? What's next?"

As we recovered in the locker room after the match, Nova asked me why, when he'd kicked me in the back of the head, I fell on my back instead of doing the forward flip that was expected. Chuckling, he said, "It looked weird." He may as well have been speaking a foreign language, because I didn't know what he was talking about. Eager to protect my reputation and shift the blame for the screw-up onto him, I quickly broke into character and said in the most condescending voice I could muster, "Because you kicked me so hard I blacked out, you jerk." (I didn't really say "jerk.") I had no idea if that was what had actually happened, but it worked because everybody laughed. Two years later I found out it was funny because it was true. When I began tracing my concussion history, I finally convinced Nova to give me his copy of the tape of the match. He knew that I was looking for that kick; he had been in denial for the last two years that the kick was any big deal. But as he handed it to me he confessed, "By the way, I kicked you so hard that I honestly thought I broke my foot." On the tape after he kicked me in the head, I froze in midair as if I'd slipped on ice.

Dr. Cantu asked if I'd felt anything strange after the match. "Yeah," I said, "but I thought it had to do with my nose."

This had been one of my first matches after a complicated surgery to replace the cartilage in my nose with plastic. I needed surgery after my face was smashed in the 2003 Royal Rumble—courtesy of the wrestler Edge.* In addition to giving me a concussion, Nova had fallen on my nose and undone the surgery—which was painful, bloody, and annoying enough to garner my full attention after the match. That made it especially easy to forget about the blackout.

"Yes, the evidence would point to that being a concussion," Dr. Cantu concluded.

"Hmm, that means I've had two concussions now," I thought. "Wait a minute . . . What if I was involved in a big collision in football, but I don't remember feeling the hit? I do remember that the sky turned orange for a few minutes."

During a preseason intersquad scrimmage in my sophomore year in college, I was on the kickoff-return team as a blocker. In 95 percent of kickoffs, the kicker sends the ball as far as he can, and a small, fast kickoff-return specialist will catch it and run it back. Unfortunately, our backup kicker was terrible, and kicked it 20 yards short—right to me. Since I was big, dumb, and slow, I just ran straight ahead. When I saw our best headhunter, Clint Kollar, coming at me, I lowered my head and ran straight for him. When I opened my eyes, I noticed that everyone was excited, but I didn't know if they were excited for me or for Clint. I didn't know whether I'd crushed him or he'd crushed me. I never felt anything. I didn't understand why they congratu-

---

*The injury wasn't Edge's fault. In fact, he probably saved me from a crushed skull by twisting his body in midair before he kicked me. My advice to the kids at home: Don't ever agree to be double-dropkicked from the top rope.

lated both of us until I saw the film the next day. The explosive hit caused us both to fall sideways, and it looked awesome on film. I distinctly remembered staggering to the sideline, taking a knee, and blinking about a thousand times to see if I could get the sky to turn from orange back to blue.

Dr. Cantu remarked, "That definitely fits in the concussion category."

"Wow, I've had three concussions," I thought.

Then I remembered another one.

"Once during the filming of *Tough Enough,* I got clotheslined in the face, the sky turned orange for a few minutes, and I was told that I acted strangely for the rest of the day. What about that?"

On the last day of *Tough Enough* practice, the students wrestled the trainers. WWE Superstar Tazz decided to rough me up a little, a common initiation into the business from a veteran to a rookie. I survived about ten legitimate kicks to the back of the head. Then he picked me up, threw me into the ropes, and tried to take my head off with a clothesline. The hit was so hard that I saw stars, but I ignored them as I spat out bits of chipped teeth. Before I knew what had hit me, I had to brace myself to land; Tazz unceremoniously threw me out of the ring between the ropes. As I sat outside the ring, I didn't realize right away that I had broken some teeth. I was just glad to be out of there. The other trainer, Al Snow, later told me that I had seemed "out of it" for the rest of that day. At the time, I wasn't worried about it. It was the last day of the competition and I still had judges to impress.

Dr. Cantu nodded and said, "Yes, that was probably . . . "

"What if I was playing football, got 'dinged' when I was blindsided by a hit, and later was told that I called people by the wrong name in the dining hall that night at dinner?"

"Yes, that . . . "

"How about being elbowed in the face during a tag-team match, spending five minutes outside the ring seeing double, and then trying to figure out where I was?" I asked. I got a scar on my cheek that time, so it was easier to verify.

"Could have been," he said.

That added up to about a half-dozen concussions from the age of 18 on—that I could remember.

"Having had multiple concussions could be the reason why you're not recovering as quickly as we'd like," said Dr. Cantu.

I asked him to explain.

Dr. Cantu told me how most concussion symptoms are transient, meaning that they don't last very long. The chart on concussion symptoms in Chapter 3 makes that point clear. The researchers went back and asked athletes which symptoms had persisted three days after the injury.

Symptom	% Reporting at Time of Injury	% of Those Reporting Symptom Three Days Later
Headache	92%	45%
Dizziness	72%	12%
Blurred vision	67%	17%
Disorientation	58%	0%
Confusion	56%	10%
Disequilibrium	44%	0%
Nausea/vomiting	39%	14%
Anterograde amnesia	31%	18%
Neck pain	31%	64%
Photophobia	31%	36%
Sleepiness	28%	60%
Fatigue	25%	33%
LOC	19%	NA
Retrograde amnesia	19%	14%
Irritability	17%	50%

Source: Guskiewicz KM, Ross SE, Marshall SW. Postural Stability and Neuropsychological Deficits After Concussion in Collegiate Athletes. *Journal of Athletic Training* 36:3 (2001): 263–373.

As the chart shows, some of the symptoms (such as disorientation) disappeared, while others (such as irritability and sleepiness) took a few days to appear.

The unique symptoms that each concussion causes can be related to the area of the brain that has been traumatized. Dr. Cantu has written, "Some symptoms relate primarily to the brainstem or dysfunction of its connections, like unconsciousness, tinnitus, lightheadedness, unsteadiness, ataxia, headache, nausea, vomiting, and incoordination. Other symptoms result from cerebral cortex dysfunction and occur acutely, including confusion, disorientation, anterograde and retrograde amnesia, decreased information processing, and short-term memory impairment. Still others may be delayed in onset, like depression, fatigue, sleep disturbance, irritability, and feeling 'foggy.'"[1] Unfortunately, this way of understanding symptoms is murky, because if the injury is "diffuse," many different parts of the brain can be injured in a single concussion, and the neurometabolic cascade can affect the function of multiple parts of the brain.[2][3]

Thus in order for Dr. Cantu and me to predict when my specific symptoms would disappear, we had to think at a more basic level. We knew that the malfunction was primarily caused by two processes, physical damage and the neurometabolic cascade. It's easy to understand why we recover from a neurometabolic cascade—eventually the ions in the brain become balanced, and blood flow returns to normal.

However, if there was physical damage, the brain doesn't return to normal in the same way; the damage is permanent.

Dr. Cantu told me, "When we say the brain has healed, the damage is permanent. However, you can return to the functional level you previously had because there are enough spare parts of the brain to take over that function. Although it's more complex than this, one way of looking at it is that we are born with millions of extra nerve cells and neurons. This explains why people can start losing them in their twenties, and still be mentally keen in their eighties. Obviously the greater number of extra cells you are born with, the greater number you can lose before you're down to a critical level—before you start to see neurologic deterioration.

"What happens with multiple head injuries is that in some instances, you lose thousands, if not more, nerve cells. Then you reach a critical limit, where you start not to have enough nerve cells to function at the level that you once did. You now pick up permanent rather than transient neurologic impairment. That's a supply-and-demand way of looking at it."

The brain uses the extra neurons to compensate, and this leads to recovery from physical damage. This is called *plasticity*. However, you eventually run out of spare parts. Using this framework, my lack of recovery could have been an indication that I had reached some sort of "critical point" where I was running low on extra neurons. With that as a possibility, Dr. Cantu attached a medical label to my predicament: "post-concussion syndrome." I was familiar with that syndrome, as it has ended many athletes' careers.

The idea that at a certain point you can no longer recover as quickly or fully from concussions is supported by a multitude of studies that show after suffering one concussion, athletes are three to six times more likely to have a second one.[4] [5] [6] [7] [8] Plus, additional concussions tend to be more severe. People with a history of concussions are between four and seven times more likely to get knocked unconscious.[9] [10] In essence, we chip away at some sort of "brain reserve."

Dr. Cantu decided to perform an MRI to see if there was any physical evidence of brain damage. I told him that I'd already had one, and it was negative.

"While it's a longshot, sometimes the evidence can take a while to appear, and sometimes you just have to know what to look for," he said.

I left the doctor's office with more answers but even more questions.

▼▼▼

A few days later, I drove back to the hospital for my second MRI in two months. The MRI process is always impersonal; you don't know the nurses and technicians, and they don't know anything about you, save for the part of your insides that a doctor wants to see. This encounter was no different. I slipped into the tube with nary a word spoken. Some people find being trapped in that tiny tube with the loud noises and vibrations of the machine claustrophobic. I've had so many MRI's over the years that I usually fall asleep. This particular morning, the technician interrupted my nap. My new habit of acting out my dreams was causing me to squirm, ruining the MRI images. When I left, I felt anxious about the test results. Yet, since I was confident they wouldn't find anything wrong, I figured the only harm done was having wasted the morning.

On my way home from the hospital, I got a phone call from a number I didn't recognize. It was the MRI technician. With a strange tension in her voice, she urged me to return the next morning for another test.

Hesitating, I asked, "Why, did something not work?"

"We'd like to take some more pictures" was all I could get her to say.

I couldn't tell if she was hiding some huge discovery that they would only tell me in person, or if she honestly didn't know why they wanted to see me again. Either way, that's a phone call you don't want to get. I got more worried when I found out that this busy MRI center (I'd had to wait over a week for my first appointment) had cleared an early morning appointment the next day.

From the moment I hung up the phone, I desperately tried to figure out what diagnosis could possibly require such an urgent second test. Scenarios ran through my mind like flash cards. The stack of cards was short, due to my lack of knowledge of the brain and my lack of imagination. I could only think of two legitimate reasons why I had to go back. Either they had made a mistake, and nothing was wrong (this is what I was hoping for) or they had found a brain tumor (this terrified me). What else could be so urgent that I had to go back to the hospital the next day, but not urgent enough that I didn't have to go that very second? I figured that a tumor would explain why my symptoms weren't going away.

I had to stop torturing myself, so I distracted myself by watching a movie, and then tried to go to bed. I figured I'd have plenty of time to make myself crazy on the 45-minute drive to the hospital the next morning. Despite my best efforts, and the usual sleeping pills, I didn't get much rest that night.

When I arrived the next morning, everything seemed eerily normal. The same nurses and technicians were there. No one was acting weird—as far as I could tell. They slid me into the tube again. There was a mirror over my head set at a 45-degree angle so I could see out past my feet—probably there for the claustrophobics. I had a good view of the technician's room, where they watch the live pictures on computer screens. In my experience, there are usually only one or two people in the technician's room. I did a quick head count. One, two, three, four . . .

"Uh, oh," I thought. "That's too many people."

In addition to the two technicians, I saw Dr. Cantu and another man wearing a lab coat. I assumed he was the doctor scrutinizing the pictures on the screens. No one had told me that all those people would be there. I don't think I was supposed to know they were there. It was just my luck that two workmen were installing new blinds over the windows that day, so the doctors were in full view. I felt a wave of nausea and started to sweat. I wanted out of the tube.

After twenty more minutes of agony, the test was over. The doctors had left, and the technicians weren't very talkative. I was told to go up to Dr. Cantu's office on the eighth floor. That hadn't been on the agenda either. Not good. When I arrived, there were four people in the waiting room, but I wasn't even given a chance to sit down. I was whisked right in to see the doc.

By this time, I think I'd stopped breathing. Dr. Cantu must have noticed, because he gave me an overly reassuring smile.

"Don't worry, you're fine."

A wave of relief swept over my body, followed by a wave of confusion. "What did you think was wrong?"

"Well Chris . . . you have a few small areas in and on the surface of your brain that show up as white spots on the MRI. Multiple white spots can be early evidence of multiple sclerosis. We had to rule that out, and we did."

"How?" I asked.

"If you had MS, you'd have a lot more of the spots."

He seemed satisfied. I was not. "Okay, then what are these spots?"

"Well, the answer is that we don't know . . . I would venture to guess they're most likely the residual evidence of tissue damage caused by impacts—concussions. But they look like they've been there for a while, so they're probably not from your latest ones."

"Does that confirm that I've had concussions that I didn't know about?" I asked.

"More than likely," he answered.

I sat back in my chair and let it all soak in. Sweet. I have dead chunks of brain from these shots I've taken. I didn't know that was even possible. By the end of the week, I would receive a physical copy of the MRI report, and would discover that "a few areas" meant five, and "small" meant as big as 4mm x 3mm on some slides. I didn't know what was considered big, but I decided that that was all the dead brain tissue I was comfortable having.

As the evidence that years of abuse had considerably damaged my brain continued to mount, I wasn't so gung-ho about returning to the wrestling ring "a week after the symptoms disappeared." Dr. Cantu had told me that it would be easy to get another concussion, and that it would probably be much worse than my latest one. If it was taking me months to get over this concussion, it could take me years to get over the next one. Or maybe I'd have the symptoms forever.

But I soon found out this wasn't the worst of my worries. There was another variable I hadn't yet thought of while planning for my return—the need to take time off between concussions. Having one more concussion would be bad, but having another one before I'd recovered from the first could be exponentially worse.

▼▼▼

I first learned about this risk when Dr. Cantu finally gave in on our "no medication" policy, and sent me to see a headache specialist. I walked from my Cambridge apartment over the Charles River to the Pain Management Clinic at Spaulding Rehabilitation Hospital. This hospital sits behind the sports arena where the Boston Celtics and Boston Bruins play. I had an appointment with Dr. Heechin Chae, the associate medical director for Spaulding's inpatient brain injury rehabilitation program, and a headache specialist. He and I bonded immediately. I had an acupuncture treatment each week. While Dr. Chae inserted the needles, I'd ask him questions about concussions, just like I did with Dr. Cantu.

Dr. Chae had so much to say that I got the feeling that he'd been waiting for someone to ask him about his experiences treating these injuries. All that year he'd been treating teenagers with post-concussion syndrome. The worst cases were kids who had received a second concussion before they had recovered from the first. He was clearly frustrated. He saw concussion treatment as a double standard, because most doctors, even neurosurgeons, treat severe brain injuries completely differently than mild brain injuries.

"I don't know how much sense that makes, because we're dealing with the same organ," Dr. Chae told me. "No cardiologist ignores a 'mild' heart attack. He doesn't say to his patient, 'Don't worry about exercise or your diet unless the heart attack is severe.' He still treats him as if he has had a heart attack. Yet we don't treat a concussion in the same way as we do a brain injury. For some reason we tell people, 'You're fine,' when we know they aren't."

Dr. Chae felt that his brain-injury treatment mantra was often lost on his colleagues. He stated, "There's nothing you can do about the initial damage from a head injury. The reason that we spend so much time, energy, and money is to *prevent further damage*. A concussion is the same principle—*it's a head injury*—but we do a terrible job preventing secondary or further injury."

If the brain receives further impacts before the chemical and metabolic fluctuations that occur after a concussion have returned to normal, the damaged brain cells, in one expert's words, "teeter on the brink," and another impact may kill brain cells that would otherwise recover.[11][12][13][14] The brain is vulnerable to permanent and severe damage during this period of days, weeks, or months, like the Death Star in the movie *Star Wars* when the deflector shield is down. (Yes, I like science fiction.)

Dr. Chae preferred a different analogy. "Imagine that the brain is a city that experiences an earthquake. The earthquake isn't bad enough to make the buildings fall down, but there is structural damage in the foundations. If there's an aftershock—and even if it's much weaker than the earthquake—the structures are more vulnerable to collapsing.

"With any kind of second earthquake, there's a risk that the buildings will fall down. I would say that's analogous to the brain. Once you damage the brain, there's some structural damage, and the brain is vulnerable to another impact. In that case, you can actually kill brain cells. Not suffering any further trauma is important because by returning to play too quickly, you expose your brain to the risk of further damage that could have easily been prevented. Sitting out allows the brain to strengthen its structures and withstand other types of injuries. Consistent with my knowledge about brain injuries in general, the second, third, and fourth injuries are a lot more detrimental to the person's long-term outcome than the first."

▼▼▼

I later found out that Dr. Chae had one patient in mind while we were discussing this little-known risk. In the fall of 2003, 12-year-old Willie Baun was a typical seventh-grader who loved to play football. His father, Whitey, was a coach of his local peewee team, and had been since Willie started playing at the age of 7. Willie's mother Becky described Willie as, "very friendly, very outgoing, very social, and good at sports. He's a 'ball' kid."

Willie got his first concussion of the season on an onside kick. He and another player went for the ball and collided helmet-to-helmet. Although Whitey was initially concerned, Willie appeared fine, and walked off the field on his own. Whitey asked one of the other coaches to check him out. The coach said that Willie was a little woozy, but fine. Willie went back in the game, but Whitey noticed by the way he was playing that something was wrong.

Whitey pulled him out, and he and Becky took Willie to the hospital after the game. The doctor said Willie had suffered a concussion and that he should take at least three weeks off, depending on when his headache went away. The headache took a full three weeks to go away, and a few days later Willie returned to the team.

Whitey remembered, "[Three weeks] seemed a little excessive at the time, but we waited, and after those three weeks, he started to play again.

For the next two weeks he seemed fine, although now I worry that he wasn't fine, but didn't want to tell me."

Five weeks after the initial concussion, Willie was taking part in an angle-tackling drill on soft ground at half speed. "Willie got hit, fell to the ground, and didn't get up," Whitey recalled, reliving every parent's worst nightmare. "I was on the other side of the field at the time. Based on the hit, I couldn't imagine that it was another concussion—he just got tapped. But when I got there I could tell something was wrong." Willie went back to the hospital, where a negative CT scan revealed it was "just" another concussion.

But after Willie returned home, things changed overnight. Willie developed amnesia. Becky couldn't believe what she saw when Willie came out of his room the next morning. "When he woke up, he didn't know the dog, and I'm not even sure he knew who Whitey and I were. As the day went along he figured out we were his parents, but I can remember him looking at me like he was trying to relearn who I was. That was so scary. He was totally dizzy, and he couldn't put one foot in front of the other. When we took him to the hospital, they said there was nothing they could do to help him."

After a few weeks, his parents tried to get Willie back into school. He started with half-days every other day, but struggled severely due to his memory loss. The school didn't think that Willie belonged in a regular classroom because he was now reading at the second-grade level. The Bauns had to convince the school that regular classes were the best thing for Willie, with the hope that he would eventually get better.

Becky often fought with the teachers. "I'd send in math work for him to do, and tell the math teacher to let him do that work instead. The teacher would call me and say, 'Well, you didn't send in work today.' I'd say, 'The work was in his pocket—he just didn't remember it was there!' Willie would wear cargo pants with four pockets. He'd have whatever he needed for each class—English, math, science and social studies—in one of the pockets. That's how he went around school. He couldn't remember where his locker was, what to carry, or what he needed for the next class. He couldn't plan ahead."

At first, Willie realized that there was something different about him. Nearly every day, he'd ask, "Why can't I do that?" Becky would have to explain to him what had happened, even though she wasn't sure if Willie would remember her explanation. "We'd keep telling him that he'd had a concussion, and the doctors were calling this post-concussion syndrome. I'd say, 'We'll go see the doctor, and we can ask questions if you want to.'"

After six months, Willie began getting his memory back, but no one can be sure if he will ever fully recover. Whitey worries that he's to blame for letting Willie return to the field too soon after the first concussion. "We don't know if the hits he took during those two weeks had something to do with what happened. I'll be driving down the road, and I'll start to think about it. I say to myself, 'I can't believe it. Why didn't you see? Why didn't you know? Did you get him back there too soon?' And the answer is . . . that although I didn't necessarily know it at the time . . . we did . . . I did. Living with that will be very difficult."

▼▼▼

After hearing Willie's story, I understood Dr. Chae's passion for requiring athletes to fully recover before going back out on the field. But while I understood the concept, I was a little hazy on the science. I turned to Dr. Hovda for an explanation.

"We think we know why brain cells die," he told me. "There are three scenarios that could explain why the cells die when the brain is hurt again during this period of time it is vulnerable.

"First, the brain gets its fuel from blood. If you open your eyes, blood flow increases to provide fuel to the area of the brain that processes vision. After a concussion, this coupling between blood flow and metabolic demand is lost. So when you stimulate the brain, the brain will still fire and ask for fuel, but the blood flow will not increase. If this happens enough, then the cells will die from cerebral ischemia, which means that the blood flow to the area isn't enough to support the demand for energy.

"The second thing that happens is that when the brain is injured from a concussion, the neurotransmitters bind on to the receptors, they change the receptors, and they stay changed for a long period of time. One of the receptors that's changed a lot is susceptible to a compound called *glutamate*. Glutamate is a neurotransmitter in the brain that is excitatory—if you excite a cell too much it will go on to die, like a seizure. If the receptors have been changed to make them much more sensitive, then just the normal stimulation from another release of glutamate—which could happen from another head injury—would overwhelm the cells, and the cells would die from what is called an excitotoxic death. This means that they fire until they die.

"The third possibility has to do with potassium being released outside the cell, causing a demand for fuel, and calcium coming inside the cell, mucking up the machinery that metabolizes fuel, called *mitochondria*. If the cell still has this high concentration of calcium, then another blow to the head will cause another flood of calcium. But this time, the calcium will overwhelm the mitochondria, and the mitochondria will die. It's similar to ingesting a toxin used in biochemical warfare, like mustard gas, that prevents the body from taking in oxygen. The cell has to make energy to survive. The brain and the body require about 116 watts of energy per hour, and if you don't make that, you start losing stuff."

The formula was relatively easy to understand. In the simplest terms, most concussions cause only temporary damage. But if an athlete continues to take shots to the head before the brain has had a chance to recover, those combined injuries cause more problems because the release of chemicals in the brain harms the interfaces between cells. That's when the athlete begins to suffer permanent damage.

Just when I thought I understood the damage caused by concussions, Dr. Chae added another process to the mix.

"While our current understanding is that a mild concussion doesn't cause brain cell death, we do believe it causes axonal degeneration. Consider the axons as 'highways' connecting the neurons. They're basically shaken by the impact. Certain types of damage trigger a cascade of events, where axons start to lose their fatty envelope. That fatty envelope is what makes the transmission of information flow properly. When you lose it, the transmission becomes much slower or gets interrupted, and there are a lot more noise factors."

Studies show concussions can change any facet of one's being that is controlled by the brain—behavior, emotion, intelligence, memory, personality, attention, mood, cognition, ability to communicate, mobility, etc. But people who are merely changed are the lucky ones. Some people don't survive that second hit.

▼▼▼

"It's called second impact syndrome, or SIS," Dr. Cantu told me. "In theory you could be at risk, but the vast majority of SIS cases occur in athletes ages 12 to 18. For some unknown reason, teenagers appear to be the most vulnerable."

I'd been reading about all these young athletes dying after they'd suffered two concussions in quick succession, and I was concerned. After all, I'd risked my own health for weeks after my concussions by trying to be a tough guy and continuing to wrestle. More importantly, I was worried that I still might be at risk in the future.

From 1980 to 1993, the National Center for Catastrophic Sports Injury Research linked seventeen deaths in football to SIS, and many more deaths have occurred since then.[15] No one is sure how and why SIS occurs, but in every case it's caused when an athlete receives a secondary head trauma before the symptoms from a first concussion have resolved. The impacts aren't always severe; sometimes they involve a hit to the chest, side, or back that causes the head to snap back.[16] Although it isn't clear what happens inside the brain of the athlete, what a coach, parent, or teammate sees from the outside is remarkably consistent. The athlete is usually dazed by the impact, but he remains alert for another fifteen seconds to a minute. Then he suddenly collapses to the ground, in a semiconscious state, with rapidly dilating pupils and a loss of eye movement. Then he stops breathing.

About half the athletes live and half die, depending on the severity of the bleeding inside the brain and the medical care the athlete receives.

On September 29, 2001, high-school football player Matthew Colby died fifteen hours after collapsing from a head injury that he had suffered on the field.[17] [18] He'd been complaining to friends of a headache that began after he'd received a hit on September 15, almost two weeks before. The headache persisted after a second game on September 21, and he complained again. The coaches became aware, he was held out of practice, and he received clearance from a doctor to play in the next game.

A forensic neuropathologist performing a microscopic examination of Colby's brain discovered evidence of brain trauma that had occurred up to two weeks prior to his death in the form of "neomembranes," which are spots of tissue formed after the dura—the membrane surrounding the brain—separates from the brain. In these cases, fragile blood vessels expand to fill the space, and while they are stretched, they have an increased risk of bursting (much like an overfilled balloon).

Those who survive the injury may never be the same. Just over ten years ago, Brad Ames of Evansville, Indiana, returned to play after ten days of rest following a concussion. He immediately got hit again.[19] The second brain injury severely damaged his ability to coordinate his muscles, so on most days it's difficult for him to speak and to be understood. His mind and personality remain intact. Some people who suffer this kind of brain injury lose their mental faculties to such a degree that they're unaware of having a problem. Brad is fully aware of what happened to him, but is powerless to do anything about it.

Brandon Schultz had a similar injury. His family sued the school district to help cover the estimated $12.6 million cost of Brandon's lifetime care.[20] His attorney said, "Brandon suffered a concussion during a game just one week prior to his tragic episode. He briefly lost consciousness, complained of headaches the week following the injury, and yet no school official referred him to a doctor. Had Brandon been required to see a doctor—what should always be a standard requirement when an athlete suffers a concussion with ongoing symptoms—we believe his SIS brain injury would never have occurred."

Brandon's mother said, "No one instructed us that a physician should clear Brandon to play. To us it was just a headache. We had no reason to believe it was anything more than that."

Brandon continues to suffer severe physical, cognitive, and psychological problems, and will always require advanced care. He's haunted by the memory of the young man he used to be. "I still think of myself as that same guy," Brandon said. "But I'm not. And I know I'm not."

▼▼▼

The more I learned about the victims of SIS, the less I felt sorry for myself and the more I began to worry about all the kids playing football. I was out of the woods; I wasn't going back to wrestling until I was symptom-free for a long, long time, and since SIS usually afflicts teenagers, I wasn't worried about dying when I did return.

But it was clear to me that these tragic injuries could be avoided if we were able to properly diagnose and treat concussions. On a personal level, I was frustrated that I didn't have the knowledge to prevent further injury to myself. It would have been nice to have avoided this whole "months of headaches and possible end of my wrestling career" thing that I was going through. But beyond any immediate thoughts of myself, I was deeply troubled by the more than 1.1 million high-school football players and hundreds of thousands of junior-high and elementary school kids who are experiencing concussions like mine, with far less support. Even with the unlimited medical budget that the WWE seemed to have for me, it took me a long time to get the information I needed. I heard a different story about concussions from nearly every doctor I saw. Willie Baun's parents, acting on the advice of three doctors, were unable to protect their son. Something wasn't adding up. Why did all these doctors have such drastically different information about this injury?

Perhaps it was related to their sources of information. As a pharmaceutical consultant for Trinity Partners, with every new project, I have to go from being a neophyte to an authority in a new area of medicine in just two to three months. I spend a lot of time at the Harvard Medical School library, reading studies that examine the current treatment methods of a specific illness, and the changes in diagnosis and treatment strategies over time. It's often my responsibility to figure out how many people have a certain illness now, and how many will have it in the future. These assignments are never easy, as the studies and data sources usually conflict. Based on who performed the study, who *paid for* the study, and how the study was designed, it's my job to determine who has the most accurate information.

It dawned on me that it might be a good idea to apply my research skills to the sports concussions universe. I thought that maybe the doctors' knowledge was inconsistent because they were getting their information from different sources, some of which may have been wrong or outdated. Perhaps they were even reading studies funded by industry, which can often make the conclusions of those studies . . . let's just say "unique." Heck, I had the time to research this—I wasn't working. It turns out that after reading just about every concussion study one could possibly get his hands on, I was proven right.

CHAPTER 5

Taking Care of the Kids

I would venture to say that I had between 15 and 18 concussions in my career. When my old teammates—or just guys in general—ask me about concussions, I ask them if they ever had one. They say, "No." I ask them if they ever saw stars flash before their eyes. And they say, "Yeah." I ask if they ever hit someone or got hit and had everything just fade into black. And they say, "Yeah." I tell them "That's a concussion." I've come to the realization that a lot of guys have suffered concussions, and the effects of concussions, and they don't even know it.

Harry Carson, 53, NFL Hall of Famer

There were times when my head hurt so bad that I felt like I was going to pass out. I was never diagnosed with a concussion; of course, I never asked the doctor to look at my head, either. It didn't mean that much to me at the time.

Brian Daigle, 26, former college football player

I've never had a concussion. I probably get my "bell rung" or get "dinged" once every game or every other game. I've never told a trainer because it doesn't really cause problems, it's just a short little bang. It's pounded in your head that you can play through anything. I just suck it up most of the time. You just have to suck it up if you want to play.

David Howard, 16, high-school junior

I'm afraid that these young kids don't really know what's going on. When they're a little dizzy, a little confused, or maybe something inside them says, "Hold it, I need to take a break," they don't tell us. So we say, "Okay Joey, get back in there. Let's go!" We think, "Let me be the macho coach. Hey kid, suck it up!" The kid doesn't tell us because he doesn't know what to say. And we don't ask the right questions to find out if he has gotten his bell rung or not.

Whitey Baun, 54, former college football player, youth football coach

I needed to take a step backward before I could move forward. My experience over the weeks since my last concussion had taught me that few doctors, let alone athletes, understood this injury well. I knew from my prior consulting experience the answers I wanted, and the answers that these doctors should have had at their fingertips, did exist somewhere in the medical literature. The original studies upon which modern head injury treatment is (or should be) based are buried inside medical journals, but not every doctor has time to keep up with them. But a researcher with enough time and motivation to read and analyze might find some answers. Time and motivation was about all I had. I started to look at the concussion studies, and I soon discovered that there's a growing body of research of varying quality on high-school, college, and professional football players. But I was frustrated to find that there wasn't a single study on football players who are middle-school age or younger. Why wouldn't we first study the players who are least able to understand or articulate this injury? I was forced to be creative to get an idea of what was happening to the little guys.

An opportunity presented itself while I was driving through Cambridge, Massachusetts, one spring afternoon. I passed a field where about one hundred kids in football helmets were practicing, and thought it would be worth my while to park my car and watch. I was surprised that kids would be practicing with helmets in June, so I was relieved to find that it was just a summer camp.

After a few minutes of watching some noncontact drills, a coach blew his whistle to end the session. I recognized him—he had been a coach of mine in college. I walked over to say hello, and as we were catching up, I told him about the project I was working on. I asked if I could talk to a few of his younger players about concussions. He made me a deal; if I would give a talk to the whole camp about football, wrestling, working hard in school, and concussions, he'd let me talk to a few seventh- and eighth-graders one-on-one.

We had a nice group chat. The kids focused on who I had beaten in the WWE, and I focused on not revealing how unimpressive that list really was. When we were done, the coach started sending kids over to talk to me.

Fourteen-year-old Patrick told me that he'd never been diagnosed with a concussion, but admitted, "Once in a while I get hit hard and my head starts throbbing. Sometimes I get a little dizzy." Thirteen-year-old Keith had a similar story. He told me, "I don't think I've ever had a 'concussion.' I know I've gotten my 'bell rung' a couple of times, and I've been pretty dizzy after some hits, but that's about it. When you get a direct hit to the head, and you get up, you get a little dizzy. My teammates have had to help me off the field before, and it's taken me a while to get my bearings back, but I doubt that I had a concussion."

Fourteen-year-old Kyle had a different story. He'd been diagnosed with a concussion the previous season. "I went down low to block someone, and his knee hit me in the head. I got dizzy, my head started spinning, and I had to go to the sideline. Then I threw up. That was pretty much a concussion, they said. That's my only serious one. Sometimes after a hit, when I go back to the huddle, I'll be weaving back and forth, but by the time we get back up to the line I'll be fine. I don't consider those concussions. But ever since I got the concussion, if I run too hard or if I get hit too hard, I start feeling dizzy and tired. Then it'll go away. It comes and it goes. It happens in anything. Say I run two miles. I'm really dizzy at the end. That didn't use to happen—it's just since the concussion."

It was clear from these short conversations that these young men were suffering concussions. So why the lack of attention from the medical community? Perhaps it's because people incorrectly assume that kids are too small and too slow to get concussions. That's what Willie Baun's mother had thought. "I didn't worry about concussions at the time because the kids were all so slow, they were all so padded, and it never seemed like they picked up enough speed to bounce off of someone with much impact."

Personally, I think that no one has looked into this simply because they believe that it would be too difficult. Youth teams don't keep medical records like the upper levels of football do, and few employ medical staff. This means that there's no free data to be had. Researchers probably think that children would be poor sources of concussion histories, as well. Many would doubt kids' ability to accurately say or even remember if they'd had a concussion. We certainly haven't provided much successful educational outreach to help kids understand or care about the concussions they may be getting; a recent study showed that over half the athletes at the University of Akron have no knowledge at all of the possible consequences following a head injury.[1] If college athletes don't think that concussions are dangerous, what hope do we have for middle-school students? Would they consider a concussion to be an event worth remembering?

With or without data, understanding what's happening to kids on the football field is an important question for the hundreds of thousands of youth football players and their parents. Unfortunately, we must learn our lessons from the groups who *have* been studied: college, high-school, and professional football players. And here, the studies paint a disturbing picture.

▼▼▼

Dr. J. Scott Delaney is a team doctor for the McGill University football and soccer teams, as well as for the professional football and soccer teams in Montreal. A specialist in emergency medicine and sports medicine, he was inspired to conduct multiple studies on the incidence of concussions in these sports because after a few years with the teams, he "was taken aback at how many player-games were lost to concussions."

"Incidence" is just a fancy word for the number of concussions that happen in a given period of time. In researching early incidence studies, Dr. Delaney would have found that the largest and best-known studies claim that approximately 5 percent of football players at the high-school and college levels get a concussion each season. According to my own research, just one study at that time had ever reported a number higher than 8 percent. The studies that have reported such low numbers have a common method—they ask athletic trainers how many concussions they treat each season.

Incidence of Concussions in Football According to Trainer Surveys

Study	Level	Percent of Players Receiving Concussion
Guskiewicz et al [2]	High school and college	5%
Barth et al [3]	College	8%
Guskiewicz et al [4]	College	6%
Zemper [5]	College	4%
McCrea et al [6]	High school	4%
Powell and Barber-Foss [7]	High school	4%

Dr. Delaney questioned that methodology. From experience, he knew that players don't always tell trainers when they've had a concussion. As he told me, "When you ask a football player if he has a headache or neck pain, he usually says, 'No.' If you ask, 'You really have no headache or neck pain?' he'll say, 'Well, just my regular headache and neck pain.' "

To get past football players' tendency to minimize their injuries at the time they occur, Dr. Delaney tried asking the players directly about their experiences after the season. In association with the Canadian Football League Players' Association, Dr. Delaney conducted a pilot study where he surveyed the athletes about their experiences with concussions in the CFL. To his surprise, the pilot study was a failure. Dr. Delaney discovered that players were unwilling to admit to concussions both on *and off* the field. He told me, "In the very first study, we asked players to write their names on the studies, so we'd know who'd returned them. When we got them back, almost no players had said that they'd ever had a concussion, with the exception of those guys who were very secure with their position on the team—like the star quarterback. The others were worried that it would get back to the GM that they were prone to concussions."

So Dr. Delaney went back to the drawing board. "We sent out the same study again, but this time we made it anonymous. When the players didn't have to worry about their answers being traced back to them the numbers went through the roof. They reported 10 to 40 times more concussions," he explained.

Dr. Delaney isn't the only researcher to make this discovery. The fact that the vast majority of concussions are never revealed to athletic trainers has been reported in multiple studies across numerous age groups. Post-season anonymous surveys of football players consistently reveal that about half suffer concussions each season, and many of them suffer multiple concussions.

Incidence of Concussions in Football According to Player Surveys

Study	Level	Incidence	Average Per Player
Langburt et al [8]	High school	47%	3.4
Delaney et al [9]	College	70%	4+
Delaney et al [10]	CFL	48%	NA
Woronzoff [11]	College	61%	NA
Gerberich et al [12]	High school	19%	NA
McCrea et al [13]	High school	15%	NA

The wide range of findings is rather easily explained by looking at the survey language. With the athletes' lack of awareness about concussions, some researchers have had to try different approaches in order to get accurate data from players. Dr. Langburt and his colleagues removed the word *concussion* from their survey. They used *head injury* instead, assuming that many athletes believe that a concussion requires a loss of consciousness. They were right to consider how the injury is labeled. One survey of college football programs found that 92 percent of athletes and coaches believe that a "bellringer" and a "dinger" are different from a concussion. Actually, they're both just slang for a mild concussion.[14] The McCrea study, which found the fewest concussions, simply asked, "How many concussions did you have?"

When I finished reading the twelve studies, I was shocked by the wide gap between these two bodies of research. No matter who was "correct," I couldn't believe that so many intelligent people could be that far off, one way or the other. When compared to a trainer-based study funded by the NCAA, Dr. Delaney's college survey would imply that only 1 out of 100 concussions is being diagnosed! He stands by his data. "We chose symptoms conservatively—these are the symptoms that you can only get from concussions. We didn't want people questioning our results."

Based on my research, my experience, and the experiences of other athletes, I have no doubt that anonymous player surveys are accurate. But I find it very strange that I'm in the minority. Dr. Delaney agrees.

"I stand on the sideline for pro football and soccer, college football and soccer, and pro boxing. When you hear some of the numbers from other studies, you scratch your head and think, 'Are they dreaming? Have they ever seen how violent this game is? Or are they just living in a lab somewhere? They can't actually believe those results.' Anybody who's been there realizes there's no way they're even scratching the surface on this."

▼▼▼

Wayne Ryan, a 31-year-old former college player, played for fifteen years without telling a trainer about his numerous concussions. "First of all, I never admitted to anyone that I'd gotten a concussion," he told me. "Even if it was pretty bad, I'd just plow right through it. The only way that I wouldn't have carried on is if I'd fallen down dead."

Wayne provided a wide range of justifications for his behavior, but his biggest motivator was pride. He told me, "I would do everything in my power to stay on the field. I didn't want to let my teammates or my school down." But Wayne also had practical concerns—he didn't want to lose his starting position. He said, "If I had a starting position, I didn't want another guy coming in and taking it. I had a responsibility to myself. I wasn't going to let anybody take what was mine."

With the help of his teammates, Wayne hid his concussions. "One of the worst ones I had was against Eastside (the high school in the movie *Lean On Me*). Their middle linebacker came in on a blitz. It was a run play, so I went at him with a full head of steam. Bing-bang—we both crumbled onto the turf. I smacked my head on the back of the turf, got up and I played through the rest of the game.

"But while I continued to play, I couldn't remember anything. I couldn't remember the snap count. My guard had to tell me what to do for every play, and sometimes had to tell me twice at the line of scrimmage. But I never told the coaches that. I only told my teammates. On the bus ride back, they made sure that I didn't fall asleep, and they worked it out so someone called me every two hours to wake me up throughout the night."

▼▼▼

As eager as Wayne's teammates were to help him hide his concussion from their coaches and trainers, I think it's safe to assume that players aren't rushing to tell adults about their injuries. If we accept that football players suffer ten to one hundred times more concussions than previously thought, it turns our understanding of these injuries on its head. If the major goal in concussion treatment is to prevent secondary impacts, we're failing.

Player surveys reveal that concussion rates at the high-school through the professional levels are similar, but this doesn't necessarily transfer to the lower levels of the game. After all, do we really believe that a 10-year-old is just as proud or has the same fear of losing his starting position as Wayne Ryan does?

Limited information from other sports gives us some guidance. One recent incidence study in taekwondo found that middle-school students suffer concussions at nearly twice the rate of high-school students.[15] That study was so surprising that it caught the attention of three members of the U.S. Congress.

In April of 2004, less than two months after that study was released, Senator James Jeffords and Representatives Henry Waxman and Jesse Jackson Jr. sent a letter to the U.S. Olympic Committee asking them to reverse a 2002 rule that allowed 12- and 13-year-olds to use full head contact in taekwondo, on the grounds that younger athletes are more susceptible to head trauma.[16] In response, the U.S. Taekwondo Union (USTU) immediately banned all head contact for competitors under 14. Suddenly under pressure not to ruin "the integrity of the sport," the USTU then *reversed* its decision one month later, reverting to the following rule:

Junior Safety Rules, Article 1B:2a

The competitor is allowed to kick to the facial area; however, the kick must be light contact with absolute control without causing an injury or excessive contact, or the appropriate penalty shall be invoked.

What is interesting about these events, regardless of the final USTU decision, is that the legislators took action because the study indicated that taekwondo competitors get concussions at a level "three times as high as the rate for college football games."[17] Of course, they were using a trainer-based study for the football comparison, thereby underestimating the incidence of concussions in high-school football by ten to one hundred times. I'm curious to see if those same congressmen will take action to change the rules of football when they realize their mistake.

Congress and the taekwondo community reacted strongly to this study because the best medical information indicates that children really are at a greater risk for concussions—and the more severe consequences that can result from them—than high school and college athletes are. Even though that groundbreaking study found that middle-school competitors suffer twice as many concussions, some researchers believe that they may have underestimated the gap between middle-school and high-school concussion rates. Dr. Paul McCrory, one of the leaders in concussion research, has written, "In broad terms, a two- to three-fold greater impact force is required to produce clinical symptoms in children compared to adults. . . . This means that if a child exhibits clinical symptoms after a head injury, then it is reasonable to assume that they have sustained a far greater impact force compared to an adult with the same post-concussive symptoms."[18] Many concussions in children don't create recognizable symptoms as they do in adults, which allows them to go unnoticed.

In addition to these concerns about our ability to diagnose concussions in children, younger athletes deserve increased scrutiny due to three major differences between a child's brain and an adult's. The first difference is biomechanical. A child's skull is thinner than an adult's, while the mass of the child's head is greater in proportion to the rest of his body. In addition, children's neck muscles—which they use to hold up their large heads—are less developed. While an adult's strong neck may act as a barrier to a concussion or to whiplash, as the neck can absorb some force before it reaches the brain, a child's large head and weak neck allow more force to reach the brain. In football, we add a heavy helmet to the already poor head/body mass ratio, further stacking the odds against children.

The second difference is that a child's brain takes longer to recover from a concussion, so that there's a longer period of vulnerability. Conventional wisdom would suggest that kids bounce back from injuries faster than adults do, but evidence indicates that the opposite is true with regards to the brain.[19] One recent study found that on average it took three days for a college athlete to regain "normal" memory function after a concussion; for high-school kids, it took seven days.[20] A separate study of over two thousand high-school football players that used sensitive computerized neuropsychological tests found that while the average recovery from a concussion took about a week, 30 percent still hadn't recovered after two weeks and 15 percent hadn't recovered after three weeks.[21] There's an absolute minimum amount of time required to legitimately recover from a concussion as well; concussed high-school kids who appeared to "recover" on the sideline and showed no visible symptoms within fifteen minutes of their concussion still showed cognitive deficits on computerized neuropsychological tests thirty-six hours later.[22] So while you may see your favorite NFL player go back into the same game after a concussion and appear to be fine, it's important to know that, according to the latest and best research, kids will take no less than thirty-six hours (and many will take half a season) to safely return to the playing field.

The third reason that concussions are more dangerous for children than for adults has to do with the inherent differences between a developing brain and a mature one.[23] Dr. Chae was the first to tell me that brain development continues well into the teen years, and a brain injury at any time can permanently hinder that development.[24] "Children are a very interesting case," he said. "We think that their brains might be more flexible, and that there may be neuron growth, but, on the other hand, they might be more susceptible to damage while they're recovering from the first injury. Because the brain is reorganizing and reformulating, any kind of injury can make that damage permanent."

Not only can an injury become permanent, but an injury can cause a child to miss critical windows of development.[25] Dr. Christopher Giza, a neurologist at the UCLA Brain Injury Research Center, has pioneered studies explaining this phenomenon. He's found that injured brains in rats never grow to their full potential.[26] [27] [28] It's been known since the 1960s that young rats reared with other rats in an enriched environment (large cages with balls, wheels, toys, and tubes) develop larger and better functioning brains than do rats reared alone in smaller, empty cages. Dr. Giza discovered that the brains of young rats that have suffered concussions don't benefit from the enriched environment. How does this research on rats translate to children? Dr. Giza said, "Maybe at 6 years of age, you can't do algebra. But if your brain doesn't grow a certain way between 6 and 15, you may never be able to do algebra very well." [29] Dr. Hovda agreed, telling me, "A brain injury during a critical window can cause retardation in a certain process as we grow up."

Dr. Giza thinks that the major cause of the developmental dysfunction may be the neurometabolic cascade, specifically the indiscriminate release of glutamate following a concussion. [30] [31] A child's brain may be up to 60 times more sensitive than an adult's to "glutamate mediated N-methyl-D aspartate (NMDA) excitotoxic brain injury."[32] [33] While normal stimulation of the NMDA receptor is essential to brain development and plasticity, Dr. Giza believes that overstimulation may cause it to malfunction, basically shutting down brain development for a critical period of time.

Study after study supports the theory that childhood brain injuries can lead to severe and permanent consequences:

1. Kids who were tested five years after suffering a traumatic brain injury (TBI) experienced a slowed growth curve in academic achievement scores, especially in reading and math. The younger the child at the time of injury, the more pronounced the deficit, even with only mild or moderate injuries.[34]

2. A study found that 43 percent of kids between the ages of 5 and 15 tested more than two years after they'd suffered a mild brain injury had behavioral or learning problems that led to their being described as having a "moderate disability." According to their parents, 21 percent also had personality changes.[35]

3. A study of memory disorders in children following TBI found that memory regarding procedures, known as implicit memory, are not often

affected, yet over half the children had trouble remembering events from the past or plans for the future.[36]

4. A study of children between the ages of 6 and 15 found that one year after traumatic brain injury, nearly half (48 percent) still suffered from psychiatric disorders that had appeared after the injury, led by attention-deficit/hyperactivity disorder (ADHD) and depression.[37]

The author of one study, Dr. Carol Hawley, noted, "It's likely that there are considerable numbers of children in the community, and back at school, who have suffered a head injury in the past and who might have subtle but important difficulties relating to that head injury."[38]

Beth Adams, a neurotrauma rehabilitation specialist, treats those children. I first met Beth in her Salem, Massachusetts, office after Dr. Cantu recommended that I see her to help with my own recovery. As time went on, I began to ask about her experiences with younger athletes. Due to her affiliation with Boston's Brigham and Women's Hospital Neurological Sports Injury Center and the Spaulding Rehabilitation Hospital Concussion Clinic, she's seen a wide range of sports concussion cases.

She's particularly concerned with football, as she has two young boys champing at the bit to play. She told me, "It's difficult to watch young Pop Warner kids out there learning how to tackle. A player gets up and is dizzy. It's unbelievable, but the coach will put the player back in because the kid is willing to shake it off. The coaches just say, 'They're young and they're learning to tackle.' I worked with one kid who got a second concussion a couple of weeks after his first. He started to have memory problems right away, but you know what? That coach told him, 'You're okay. You seem to be aware and alert. Get back in there.' "

As I was researching undiagnosed concussions, I called Beth to ask what she thought was happening at the junior-high and elementary-school levels. She told me, "Concussions often go undetected and undiagnosed because kids don't know what they're feeling. They fall a lot when they're young, and they learn to just dust themselves off and get back up. I fundamentally believe that kids aren't really able to understand these injuries until they're in high school, but by high school, for many of them, the problem has already developed." I thought that was a curious way to put it.

"What do you mean 'the problem has already developed?'" I asked.

"I believe that there could be a lot of kids who are misdiagnosed and medicated for various behavioral or emotional problems that may actually be head-injury related. Not many studies have looked at that. My guess would be that there are kids, and you and I can probably remember who these kids were in school—the class clown, the kids who got into trouble—who had had blows to the head that resulted in classic post-concussion symptoms. They were 'all over the place,' hyperactive, distracted; if someone came in the room they couldn't stay focused. I'm working specifically with kids who are labeled as aggressive, or as having ADD. Many of these kids may have been hit at a particular age, but the hit was never addressed as a concussion. Now these kids are identified as 'problematic' or 'troublesome.' Sure, they might have ADD. I'm not saying they couldn't. Or, the problem could be purely behavioral or a learning disability—but I fundamentally believe that, for some of these kids, their difficulties could be traced back to a blow to the head."

One of Beth's roles is to integrate kids who've had multiple concussions back into school. She spends much of her time working with the parents and schools to set up special strategies for the child. "For the kids who have developed behavior problems, I often have to talk to the teachers and the special education program staff. I say, 'It's the hit to the head that's forcing the hyperactivity. He might require medication to calm his hyperactivity and the thoughts that are racing through his head, or he might require a program to get him to focus and stay attentive.' I see the classic dizziness and headaches, but I also see a kid who can't sit still in a chair."

A unique subset of Beth's patients includes children who already had attention deficit disorders, behavioral disorders, or learning disabilities before their concussions. Studies show that these kids tend to have more severe problems after they suffer a concussion than normal children do, as if their brains aren't able to respond as well. [39] [40] [41] [42] [43] [44] [45] Beth told me, "The parents are saying, 'The kid is just 'fill in the blank.' If the child has ADD to begin with, he's going to have an exacerbated version of ADD. The parents think that the child is just mushrooming for some reason, maybe because he's upset that he can't go back to football. However, this is really the brain's way of responding to the injury."

It's obvious to me that more attention needs to be paid to young children on the football field. But so far, we've only explored what happens to these young players in the short term. The latest and most interesting research—especially to someone who has ever suffered a concussion—concerns what will happen to those kids when they grow up.

CHAPTER 6

Lost Memories

I'm a big Cowboys fan. I see someone like Troy Aikman having to stop his career early, and I start to think, "What are these guys defining as a concussion?" when they only have three, four, or five concussions and they're ending their careers. That makes me think, "Were those things that I had concussions?" If so, I think about how many concussions I've had. Yet I still kept playing. I certainly wasn't signing million dollar contracts—I played because I loved it.

Frank Volpe, 26, former college football player

I've heard about concussions triggering Alzheimer's and some things, but nothing in real detail. To be honest, some of this stuff was presented to me, and was incorporated into my decision to retire. Some of the research is still pretty gray, and they don't know for sure, but I thought it was strong enough to make it in my interest to retire. Did it help me in my retirement? Sure, but those are all things I'd wish I'd known prior. Right now, a lot of these things are coming out after the fact, but they need to come out before the fact.

Merril Hoge, 41, nine-year NFL veteran

Other than being susceptible to further concussions, I don't know the long-term effects of having concussions. I feel like I'd only want to know that after I stopped playing. I wouldn't have wanted to know before, because it might have scared me a bit.

Ray Hill, 21, college football player

Surprisingly, the first person to tell me that there are serious, long-term consequences to concussions wasn't a doctor. Even though they were treating me for post-concussion syndrome, the doctors didn't seem to believe that telling me was their role. Instead, I heard it from former Chicago Bear Dan Jiggetts, while we were at a black-tie dinner. My experience makes me feel confident that doctors aren't telling other athletes and parents about the long-term consequences, either. Unfortunately, there isn't a lot of information on the long-term effects for children who've suffered concussions, because there are no studies that have tracked youth football players over the course of their lives. Even the information on professional athletes is limited. However, when we combine the studies from multiple sports, the picture becomes clearer.

Soon after Jiggetts tipped me off, I saw a possible connection between football and dementia while watching ESPN late one night. Tom Rinaldi was discussing the plight of former Baltimore Colts tight end John Mackey. The second tight end ever admitted to the NFL's Hall of Fame, Mackey was the first president of the newly unified NFL-AFL Players Association, and had made history as the first player to fight the NFL's restrictive free-agency and salary rules. It was his lawsuit against the NFL in 1973 that led to the free agency that football players enjoy today.[1] Now he fights another battle—with dementia.

Mackey, now 64, was diagnosed with fronto-temporal dementia (FTD) five years ago. He had begun a steady cognitive decline, which included erratic behavior, memory loss, and indifference to finding a job. After watching the program, I decided to contact Mackey's wife Sylvia to try to learn more about his situation. A mutual friend gave me her cell phone number, but warned me that if she didn't answer, I would probably have to try again until I got her on the phone. When Sylvia travels for work, John calls her and leaves messages. But he forgets that he's called, so he calls over and over again until he fills up her voicemail's memory.

When I did finally reach Sylvia, she'd just returned home from an FTD conference, where she'd learned that her husband's neurological disease could be related to prior head injuries. Experts at the conference had said that among former athletes, football players and boxers are most likely to suffer FTD. FTD is caused primarily by damage to the frontal lobe, the area of the brain behind the forehead; some doctors believe that the unique pounding that football players take to this area may play a role in their developing this disease.[2] While it's not known how many concussions John Mackey has suffered, as a player he was known for his toughness and durability. He never shied away from taking a hit, and only missed one game in ten seasons.

Sylvia began to realize something was wrong with John when he began dressing oddly and watching the Weather Channel for hours on end. He refused to read their regular mail, but answered all the sweepstakes mail. He started keeping detailed records of when he expected to receive winner checks, which would never arrive. The final straw for Sylvia came when she overheard him on the phone telling someone that his sister wasn't married. His sister had been married for quite a while. In fact, it was a memorable relationship because her husband was fifteen years her senior and their marriage had caused considerable drama within the family. When John hung up the phone, Sylvia confronted him. John couldn't remember his sister's husband's name—or anything else about him.

Sylvia took him for an evaluation. When they were given the diagnosis of fronto-temporal dementia, she finally understood why the man she had been married to for so many years had been fading away. Her husband had been replaced by someone who couldn't remember what had happened five minutes ago, who was prone to irrational mood swings, and who now often swore at her in public.

Sylvia says that their relationship has now become more of an attachment, much like a child to a mother. Sylvia is now John's caregiver, and he depends on her physical presence. But she has had to go back to work as a flight attendant to support them, so she's away from home a lot. John attends a daycare facility that costs $1,500 a month, but he has become prone to aggression, so the facility has recommended that he be moved to a second facility—at a cost of $10,000 per month.[3] John currently receives an annual pension of about $24,000. Sylvia claims that if football were determined to be the cause of his dementia, he would receive a special disability pension that starts at $110,000. "That would make all the difference in the world to me," she said.

Sylvia puts on a very strong front. However, she's worried that eventually John will be left alone with no one to care for him. Sylvia expects that John's remaining years will follow an Alzheimer's-like pattern. She's been told that he'll become incontinent, and then won't be able to walk. The last progression will be that he won't be able to eat because he will have forgotten how to swallow. There is no way for her to know when that day will come.

▼▼▼

While one study found that people who have suffered head injuries are 3.3 times more likely to develop FTD, the challenge of John Mackey's situation is that, while he is alive, it's almost impossible to know whether his dementia was caused by head injuries, or if it was just random bad luck.[4] Because of his condition, we can't ask him what kind of concussions he may have experienced decades ago, nor is there any definitive test he can take that doesn't involve looking directly at his brain.

But we do know that multiple studies have found connections between head injuries and various neurological disorders like Alzheimer's disease, FTD, memory problems, and cognitive impairment.[5] [6] [7] [8] [9] [10] [11] One study followed more than 1,200 people who had suffered traumatic brain injuries between 1935 and 1984. The study found that, while the number of people who developed Alzheimer's disease was not higher than expected, a head injury led to an earlier onset of the disease by eight years. [12]

It takes a small leap of faith to apply head-injury research from the general population to a specific group such as football players. On the surface, a concussion that an athlete receives—especially an athlete whose face is protected by a football helmet—seems minor when compared to a head injury that occurs to someone who is in a car accident or who falls down a flight of stairs. But appearances can be deceiving. A football concussion, although it may not cause bleeding and rarely requires an ambulance, is at least as significant as that concussion that was sustained in a car accident, if not more so, because the athlete is more likely to experience secondary impacts.

The evidence is mounting that seemingly minor concussions have immediate and permanent negative consequences, and may possibly cause neurodegenerative processes to be set in motion much sooner than expected. A 1999 study was among the first to quantify that damage in *active* athletes. It discovered that suffering two or more prior concussions is associated with long-term impairment in the speed of information processing and executive functioning (which includes abilities such as planning and organization).[13]

Two other studies have found a similar pattern—that just two concussions can cause measurable permanent damage to young athletes. It's common knowledge that athletes who have suffered a recent brain injury tend to perform poorly on neuropsychological tests. However, these studies found that athletes who hadn't suffered a recent concussion, but had received two concussions in their lifetime, show the same neuropsychological deficits as recently concussed players.[14] [15]

While that research is both groundbreaking and sobering, it still doesn't directly explain the correlation between concussions in youths and dementia in adults. But thanks to a group of visionary doctors and researchers, that connection is becoming clearer. In the late 1990s, Frank Woschitz, formerly of the NFL Players Association, brought together Dr. Julian Bailes, a former neurosurgeon for the Pittsburgh Steelers, Kevin Guskiewicz, PhD, a former Steelers athletic trainer, and others to investigate the full spectrum of physical and mental challenges that face retired athletes. One area they focused on was head injuries. Dr. Guskiewicz explains, "When we began this project, we were very interested in the suspected decline of retired players who have had concussions. For years there's been this notion that 'clearly there has to be a link' between concussions and both Alzheimer's disease and the Parkinson's-like dementia of a Muhammad Ali. Yet there was very little substantiated research, so we began looking into it through self-reported data." Dr. Guskiewicz emphasizes that self-reported data, which is based on the memory of an individual, is not as strong as what is called "prospective data," where the researchers follow a group of people over time. However, since no long-term prospective data exists, we'd have to wait fifty years for the results of that kind of study. Right now, self-reported data is the best information we have.

Self-reported or not, the data that came out of this group's survey is astonishing. They studied more than 2,500 of the 3,700 or so retired NFL players who are alive today. Over 60 percent of former NFL players report that they suffered a concussion in their career, and 24 percent report that they suffered three or more. Compared to the self-reported incidence numbers in the last chapter, those totals might seem low. Yet to truly understand these numbers, we have to look more closely. Some of the older players surveyed may not understand the modern definition of concussion. This would have lead them to underestimate the number of concussions they'd had. The data indicates this was likely the case, as half of the ex-NFL players who suffered a concussion said that they'd been knocked unconscious at the time. In one of his studies, Dr. Delaney found that only 5 percent of concussed players had been knocked out.[16] If we assume that both groups were knocked unconscious at the same rate, the NFL group underreported the number of concussions they suffered by ten times.

But no matter how the concussions are counted, the trends in the data are telling. As a group, NFL players had a 37 percent greater risk of developing Alzheimer's disease than did other males of the same age in the United States.[17] Retired players reporting three or more concussions were five times more likely to be diagnosed with mild cognitive impairment (MCI) than were retired players who reported never having had a concussion.[18] In addition, their rate of "significant memory problems" increased with each concussion.

Number of Concussions	Self-Reported Memory Problems	Spouse/Relative Reported
0	5.2%	8.0%
1–2	8.8%	11.0%
3	17.4%	15.0%

MCI is a difficult medical diagnosis to understand. In everyday living, it may be characterized by "forgetting or confusing names, telephone numbers, directions, conversations, and daily events."[19] Dr. Guskiewicz explained, "The best way to describe MCI would be as a precursor to Alzheimer's disease. Not everybody who has mild cognitive impairment converts to Alzheimer's disease, but a certain unknown percentage does." In a separate study of a normal population, researchers discovered that a previous head injury is the second-strongest indicator of mild dementia, with mercury exposure being the first. (I find this interesting because the Mad Hatter from *Alice in Wonderland* has always been one of my favorite characters. He was so named by Lewis Carroll because mercury was once used in hat manufacturing, causing many "hatters" to develop psychosis from mercury poisoning.[20])

Pete Cronan was one of those players surveyed. I met Pete at a cardiovascular screening for retired players sponsored by the NFL Players Association. I'd been invited to the screening by a prominent doctor who supported my research, so that I could meet and learn about the experiences of players just like Pete. Now 51 years old, Pete was an All-American at Boston College and played nine seasons with the Seattle Seahawks and Washington Redskins, winning a Super Bowl with the Redskins.

Pete was willing to share his experiences with me partially because he's concerned about what's happening to him. He admitted, "Over the last four or five years, my short-term memory seems to be eroding. My wife has noticed it. I'll give you an example. When I was in college, I vividly remember being able to walk into a room, meet twenty-five people, and remember their names at the end of the night. Now if I don't write a name down, it's gone.

"Very frequently, I think, 'I have to go into the garage to get something.' I walk into the garage, and I won't remember what the hell I went in there for. I've had to become a creature of habit because of my memory. I put my wallet, car keys, and cell phone in the same place so I don't have to think about where they are. If I don't, I don't even know where to start to look. If my phone isn't where I normally put it, I immediately think, 'Okay, it must be in the slacks I wore last night.' Then I have to concentrate on what I wore the night before. 'What the hell did I do? Where did I go? What did I have for dinner? Who was I with?' And it's happening more often."

Based on what he's learned from the media, Pete is worried that his current memory problems may be linked to seven serious concussions that he remembers getting while playing football. "I had two in high school, two in college, and three in the NFL," he said. "My freshman year at BC, against Pittsburgh, I got a concussion when my head bounced on the Astroturf. Right after the injury a guy asked me, 'What day is it?' I used to play high-school football on Sundays, so I said, 'Sunday.' Of course it was Saturday, so he said, 'You should sit down.' In 1975, I got a concussion where I actually split open my helmet. It was a short yardage play. He didn't get the yards, but I was out of it for about four hours. I've been told that I was walking around, talking and coherent, but I had no short-term memory."

Like me, Pete is aware that saying he has had seven concussions is arbitrary. "The actual number of concussions depends on the level of severity you're talking about," he said. "There is no real clear definition of a concussion. I categorize my concussions as a loss of memory and a loss of awareness of where I was. How many times did I hit guys, get up from the pile, see stars, and feel a little lightheaded? I bet I had a hundred of those. I think that's a much more common occurrence than the full-blown blackout. But if that's your definition of a concussion, then it's happening during every play."

From our discussion, it was obvious that Pete has a very clear idea of how his concussions could accelerate the onset of Alzheimer's disease. "There's some Alzheimer's in my family, but it usually comes on when a person is in his mid-seventies. If I already have a genetic predisposition, and I've compounded the problem because of concussions, it may come on in my mid-fifties instead.

That's a legitimate concern of mine, because too often I find myself scratching my head and thinking, 'Jesus, I can't remember anything like I used to.'"

It would be rare for Pete to develop MCI in his late forties. In a normal (non-head-injury) population, the prevalence of MCI is approximately 1 percent at age 60, and may be as high as 42 percent at age 85.[21] The annual conversion rate from MCI to full-blown Alzheimer's disease probably ranges from about 1 percent at age 60 to 11 percent at age 85, although some studies have found much higher rates. [22] [23] [24] [25] [26] [27]

▼▼▼

While Pete Cronan has largely kept his concerns to himself, another former linebacker has been outspoken about his neurological issues that he believes began while he was playing football. Harry Carson played inside linebacker for the New York Giants for thirteen seasons (1976–1988), was selected to nine Pro Bowls, and was inducted into the Hall of Fame in 2006. Harry was known for his punishing hits. Watching football as a child on Sundays, I thought that New York Giants Lawrence Taylor, Carl Banks, and Harry Carson were the most intimidating linebacking corps in the league. And for a guy who grew up in Chicago in the mid 1980s, that's no small statement. I'm lucky to have a friend who is close with a business partner of Harry's, and Harry was gracious enough to accept my call.

Harry spoke to me as one former football player to another. "I would venture to say that I had between fifteen and eighteen concussions in my career. They weren't the kind to knock me out on the field. Instead, I'd see stars, or everything would fade to black. You know that kind." Carson was diagnosed with post-concussion syndrome two years after retiring.

He started to notice changes while he was working as a television color commentator. "I would lose my train of thought on the air and feel anxious," he said. "I was sensitive to bright lights at night; I was sensitive to a lot of noise, especially screaming kids. Sometimes I had trouble with word retrieval. Sometimes I had bouts of depression."

That last comment surprised me. I'd been depressed since my injury, but I thought it was caused by my headaches and by the fact that I could no longer wrestle. But research indicates that depression may be directly related to head injuries. [28] [29] [30] [31] The Center for the Study of Retired Athletes found that the rate of depression among ex-NFL players reporting three or more concussions was more than triple the rate of those without concussions.

Number of Concussions	Current or Former Bout with Depression
0	6.6%
1–2	9.7%
3 +	20.2%

Eighty-seven percent of the former NFL players who report having suffered from depression at some point in their lives were currently suffering from it at the time they filled out the survey, and 46 percent were being treated with antidepressant medication. Seventy-six percent said that depression "often" or "sometimes" "limits their activities of daily living." And the former football players' frequency of "feeling sad, nervous, or under stress," correlated strongly with their concussion histories.

Number of Concussions	"Sometimes" or "Often"
0	24%
1–2	33%
3	49%

Studies of multiple populations have detected a link between head injuries and depression, even among World War II veterans who suffered both combat and noncombat head injuries during the war.[32]

Harry is keeping a positive attitude. "It's just one of things that you have to manage, and then you move forward. I sort of live in the moment," he said. "I'm very cognizant of where I am right now. You never really know when it's your time, you know? So you might as well just enjoy your life as best as you can and not worry about what lies down the road."

There is much less long-term research on other consequences of head injuries, such as attention deficit disorders, emotional disorders, headaches, or personality changes. Those links may be better clarified some day. But for at least two players, the research has come too late. In 2002, NFL Hall of Famer Mike Webster died at age 50. His autopsy revealed that he suffered from a degenerative neurological disease caused by repeated head trauma. In 2005, Webster's former teammate Terry Long died at age 45. His autopsy revealed that he suffered from the same neurodegenerative ailment.

Harry Carson feels that in some small way he contributed to one of these landmark cases. "Mike Webster, who played for the Steelers, would come out to block me and I'd give him a forearm shiver to the head or to the face that would lift him up. When I was popping him, trying to defend myself and get him off of me, I didn't realize that I was causing him damage. I didn't realize it until Mike passed away in 2002. It's my understanding that Mike was diagnosed with a neurological problem."

What happened to the brains of Mike Webster and Terry Long may hold the key to my future, and to the futures of millions of football players.

CHAPTER 7

Two Autopsies

We ought to be talking about some of the things that are happening to us now. I'm sure they're not isolated events. That's one of the reasons all those guys showed up at the health screening put on by the NFL Players Association. We want to know what the hell is going on.

Pete Cronan, 51, nine-year NFL veteran

I was talking to a friend whose father played for Boston College. He remembers having multiple concussions, and he's starting to have some memory problems now. He's wondering if the problem stems from football. There are so many professional football players who are breathing, and look fine, but they have so many internal injuries. You have to read the obituaries to get the real story.

Whitey Baun, 54, former college football player, youth football coach

I can't imagine what it would be like to have depression that's caused by getting concussions. I don't think I want to know. Right now, I'm having fun playing. I'm going to keep doing what I'm doing. But should I be thinking like this? I'm not too sure.

Steve, 16, high-school football player

The image of NFL Hall of Famer Mike Webster playing center for the Pittsburgh Steelers is permanently etched in the memory of any serious football fan. Although I was only 12 years old when he retired from football, I clearly remember him as the player who never wore sleeves under his uniform, even in sub-freezing temperatures. His pale, oversized biceps hunched over the football always stood out on television; they were the calling card of a man whom many considered to be the toughest player in all of football.

Mike Webster played in the NFL for seventeen years, fifteen of those for the Pittsburgh Steelers. At one point, he started in 150 consecutive games.[1] With four Super Bowl rings, seven All-Pro seasons, and nine Pro-Bowl selections, his success on the field is virtually unmatched. Yet Mike Webster didn't find the same success off the field. After his premature death, he became a focus of the media once again.

When he passed away in September 2002, at the age of 50, the Associated Press reported, "The Steelers initially said that Webster died of a heart attack but later declined to comment. Webster was diagnosed with brain damage in 1999, an injury caused by all the years of taking shots to the head. Webster's doctors said several concussions damaged his frontal lobe, causing cognitive dysfunction. The progressively worsening injury caused him to behave erratically, and Webster briefly was homeless, sleeping in bus stations several times when he could not find somewhere to stay."[2]

Most newspaper accounts didn't capture just how difficult life had become for Mike Webster after football, but sportswriter Greg Garber did.[3] According to Garber, as Webster's mental capacity waned, he was involved in a series of failed businesses that left him broke and homeless. At times he took a laundry list of drugs: Prozac for depression, Paxil for anxiety, Ritalin or Dexedrine to keep calm, Klonopin to prevent seizures, and Eldepryl, a drug indicated for patients who suffer from severe Parkinson's disease.

By 1997, he told a doctor that his daily headaches were "blowing the top of his head off." He would ask his children to use a black Tazer gun to stun him into unconsciousness so he could sleep. His arrest for forging Ritalin prescriptions had a morose back story. His doctor had given him a pad of signed, blank prescriptions because Webster moved a lot and often lost his pills—a result of his homelessness and memory impairment. His rare income usually came from autograph signings, and he sent most of his money to his wife and four children. He was offered assistance from many former teammates, and for a short time was supported by Pittsburgh Steelers' owner Dan Rooney, but Webster was too proud to accept their charity. Instead, he tried to come up with new business plans that would put him back on his feet. Sadly, he no longer had the ability to see any of those plans through.

Before his death, people who knew of Mike Webster's deteriorating mental health were left to speculate if it was related to his football career. After his death, that speculation was put to rest.

▼▼▼

Dr. Bennet Omalu is a neuropathologist with the Allegheny County medical examiner's office in Pittsburgh, Pennsylvania. He met Mike Webster for the first time the day after Mike died. "I was watching ESPN the morning after he died," he says. "Everyone was battering him: talking about how he died poor, how he didn't manage his resources well, etc. It struck me, because I knew that long-term play in contact sports can have adverse effects.

"I came to work and found Mike Webster's embalmed body on the autopsy table. I asked why he was in our office, and I was told that his physician had written 'chronic concussive brain injury' on the death certificate, which implies that an element of trauma contributed to his death. I began by removing his brain; I am a board-certified neuropathologist as well as a forensic pathologist and epidemiologist. I subjected his brain to very extensive analysis. I confirmed that he had structural damage to his brain consistent with chronic traumatic encephalopathy (CTE), which is often described in boxers. This was an important finding, so we published it."

When Dr. Omalu's paper was published in the prestigious medical journal *Neurosurgery*, it sent shockwaves through the medical community.[4] While chronic traumatic encephalopathy is well-established in boxing, Dr. Omalu's diagnosis was the first case of CTE ever found in a former professional football player. CTE is also known as dementia pugilistica, or "punch drunk" syndrome, but may be more accurately described as chronic traumatic brain injury (CTBI). A 1969 study found that approximately 20 percent of boxers eventually develop CTE, and many believe that it's the cause of Muhammad Ali's very public neurological decline.[5]

The symptoms of CTE and Alzheimer's disease are similar, and include cognitive impairment, parkinsonism, a loss of coordination and balance, and behavioral changes.[6][7] Studies in boxing have revealed that the risk of CTE increases with the number of boxing matches, a history of knockouts (KOs) or technical knockouts (TKOs), punches taken, or simply being a bad boxer. [8][9][10][11] Interestingly, one study of boxers between the ages of 30 and 49 found an incredibly strong correlation between CTBI and career length.[12]

Years of Experience	Percent with CTBI
Fewer than 5 years	1%
6 to 10 years	14%
More than 10 years	25%

That lends credibility to the idea that it's not only elite athletes who are at risk, but simply any athlete who has played a high-risk sport for a long time.

An examination of the wealth of literature that exists on this subject reveals that the medical community appears to be moving toward a consensus on what causes this long-term neurological decline. But since this condition is difficult to understand, I asked the expert, Dr. Omalu, to explain it to me in simple terms.

"CTE is very similar to Alzheimer's," he said. "When you have shearing forces [stress on the connections between neurons], there is disruption of what we call the skeleton of the nerve fiber, which are proteins. The nerve cell makes an attempt to reconstitute itself. Over the years, the nerve cell loses its ability to hold these proteins together. Now these proteins start becoming redistributed in the brain abnormally. Certain proteins, specifically beta amyloids beta and tau, will accumulate and take on abnormal shapes and forms in brain cells, and these brain cells begin to die. That is what I see in the brain."

Study after study reveals this pattern—traumatic brain injury causes beta amyloid and tau proteins to break away, creating "senile plaques" and "neurofibrillary tangles" (NFTs).[13][14][15][16][17][18] Senile plaques and NFTs have been found in the normal head-injury population, and specifically, in the boxing population.[19][20]

The beta amyloid plaques are believed to accumulate in the ends of damaged axons, and from there are released into other areas of the brain.[21] Axonal swelling and disconnection appears to be a process that persists for at most a few months,[22][23] but in animal studies the progressive loss of white matter of the brain as a direct result of axonal injury can span half a lifetime.[24] Researchers believe that a similar process happens in humans, which would explain why brain injuries can continue to affect people decades after the event.

The amount of plaques and NFTs that are created is logically linked to the severity of the injury. Some studies have found that after a single mild traumatic brain injury, no increase in beta amyloid or tau particles is detectable. Yet, multiple mild traumatic brain injuries do begin this process.[25][26] In a sport like football, where the evidence shows that multiple mild brain injuries are common, this is a very important discovery.

Dr. Omalu continued, "[The process] starts specifically in the frontal lobe. One of the clinical manifestations is a loss of executive function—such as business decisions, complex brain functions. It can also manifest itself as depressive disorder—as it did in Mike Webster."

Senile plaques and NFTs are more widely known as the hallmarks of Alzheimer's disease, so I was compelled to ask Dr. Omalu how he knew Mike Webster had had CTE and not a standard case of Alzheimer's disease.

He answered confidently, "This was not Alzheimer's disease because the topography of CTE is distinct." After doing my research, I knew that by 'distinct topography,' he meant that the distribution of senile plaques and NFTs within the brain is different. In Alzheimer's disease, they appear predominantly in the deep layers of the brain. In CTE, they're concentrated in the superficial layers—near the surface of the brain.[27] To a neuropathologist performing an autopsy, they are clearly distinct diseases.

▼▼▼

When Mike Webster died in 2002, very little was known about the long-term effects of sports concussions. Chance brought Dr. Omalu into this growing area of research. Inspired by his findings, he proposed new studies and sought the cooperation of NFL doctors. He recalls, "Our proposition was that 'we have just found this, let us all come together as scientists in co-operation with the NFL to study this newly identified disease.' One of my mentors, Dr. Steven DeKosky, chairman of the department of Neurology and the director of the Alzheimer's Disease Research Laboratory here at the University of Pittsburgh, sent a letter to the NFL Hall of Fame. Our proposition was, 'Since the Hall of Famers are a small, identifiable cohort of re-tired players, let us study them, perhaps having them come to Pittsburgh every six months for neuropsychiatric testing and MRI's. When they die, we'll look at their brains directly. Maybe, over the next ten or twenty years, we can learn what this disease is all about.' The NFL never responded to our two letters."

But that wasn't the end of the story for Dr. Omalu. Nearly three years later, he showed up at work and found another former Pittsburgh Steelers offensive lineman on his table. In June 2005, Terry Long, age 45, was found unconscious at his home. He died at the hospital hours later. An initial autopsy was inconclusive, but further examination of his brain revealed that, like Mike Webster, Terry Long had also suffered from CTE. Dr. Cyril Wecht, the Allegheny County coroner and one of the most well-known forensic pathologists in the world, reviewed Dr. Omalu's findings and noted, "[CTE is] a general term that we would use to denote changes in the brain of a degenerative nature. These changes can be from one intensely traumatic injury, or they can be from repetitive and cumulative injuries, which is what we believe happened here."[28] Months later, further tests revealed that Terry Long had committed suicide by drinking antifreeze.[29]

Toward the end of his life, Long was making poor decisions, indicating his brain may not have been functioning as well as it once had. Three months before his death, he was indicted by a federal grand jury on charges of fraudulently obtaining loans for a chicken-processing plant. Prosecutors alleged that in 2003 he had burned down the plant for the insurance money. He had filed for Chapter 11 bankruptcy protection just days before his death, estimating that he was more than $1 million in debt.[30]

Incidence studies like Dr. Delaney's tell us that it's very unlikely that Terry could have played for so many years without suffering multiple concussions. Dr. Omalu and his colleagues attempted to do their due diligence and piece together Terry's head-injury history, despite the fact that most concussions are never reported and therefore don't appear in medical records. "We did a postmortem psychological autopsy on Terry Long, which means that we interviewed his next of kin, his wife. She told us, 'Most of the time he would come home after playing, grab his head, and say, 'Wow, it hurts really bad.'"

When the Allegheny County medical examiner's office publicly announced that CTE was a contributing factor in Long's death, it was national news. But that was only the beginning. The next morning, Dr. Omalu picked up the newspaper to find his name being dragged through the mud by the Pittsburgh Steelers team neurosurgeon, Dr. Joseph Maroon.

Dr. Maroon had told the newspapers, "I think the conclusions drawn here are preposterous and a misinterpretation of facts. I think it's fallacious reasoning, and I don't think it's plausible at all. To go back and say that he was depressed from playing in the NFL, and that that led to his death fourteen years later, I think is purely speculative."[31] [32] This was a strong and surprising reaction to the medical examiner's report considering the wealth of evidence supporting Dr. Omalu's opinion.

Dr. Maroon's credibility was hurt, however, when he added, "I was the team neurosurgeon during [Long's] entire tenure with the Steelers, and I still am. I re-checked my records; there was not one cerebral concussion documented in him during those entire seven years. Not one."[33] [34]

Dr. Omalu said, "While he was trashing me in the newspaper, saying we were fallacious and that this was bad science, Joseph Maroon said that Terry

Long had no documented evidence of concussion. So, he's saying that if the concussion wasn't documented, it didn't exist. That's naïve. He even said that people who play football are not subjected to any form of significant concussive brain injury. That's absolutely ridiculous. I don't know what his problem is.

"But as divine providence would have it, I came across a letter in Long's record written by Dr. Maroon. The letter asked that Terry Long be suspended from play for two weeks because of a concussive brain injury." The letter, dated December 22, 1987, stated that Long had become lightheaded, dizzy, and confused, and walked with an unsteady gait after a head-on collision with a Houston Oilers player.

But that was only the beginning of NFL-affiliated doctors' attacks on Dr. Omalu's conclusions. Dr. Omalu confessed, "It was never my goal to go after the NFL. But to my utter disappointment and amazement, its response has been very negative. The NFL's mild traumatic brain injury committee actually wrote a very nasty letter to the journal *Neurosurgery*, requesting that our paper [on Mike Webster] be retracted. A member of the editorial board of *Neurosurgery* was appointed as the arbiter to review the stipulations and propositions of the NFL and our propositions and rebuttal. The editorial board strongly believed that there was some scientific truth in our paper, especially since we were simply calling for further research, not drawing any conclusions. The editorial board published both letters and made a judgment strongly in our favor, actually admonishing the mTBI committee of the NFL."

I was shocked that the NFL doctors had made such a bold attack. From the research I had read, the Mike Webster paper seemed like the logical progression of decades of research. Dr. Omalu read my mind. "That's another problem we had with the NFL. It's not like this paper is coming out of the deep blue sea," he said "There are antecedents. There are hundreds, if not thousands, of papers out there pointing to this trend! It's established that people in contact sports like ice hockey, soccer, boxing, rugby, and football manifest long-term neuropsychiatric decomposition. This was just the very first time that it had been discovered in an NFL player."

Dr. Omalu still has high hopes that the NFL will come around. "This could be handled in a very brilliant way such that the NFL wouldn't be a victim of circumstance," he said. "But it needs to acknowledge the problem and fund the right studies. The NFL's negative response gives the impression that it has always been aware of this but has hidden it from the public, just like the cigarette manufacturers."

When I began this journey—after my last concussion—I shared Dr. Omalu's optimism that the NFL would aggressively seek the answers to the many questions about concussions plaguing this sport. But based on the NFL's actions over the last decade, I'm no longer so optimistic.

CHAPTER 8

What Is the NFL Doing?

One year Paul Tagliabue, NFL Commissioner, was interviewed on concussions by reporters at the Super Bowl, and he says something like, "Worrying about concussions is a function of pack-journalism."

We expect a player in his 40s to come out of the game with aches and pains that maybe prevent him from picking up his child. But not to be able to identify that child is an entirely different matter.[1]

Leigh Steinberg, NFL agent

Some football trainers send people who have been unconscious back into the game. What is it going to take to get these guys on board?[2]

Dr. James Kelly, neurologist

I think the NFL will always look for a way to deny, deny, and deny. They want no part of [the Mike Webster case] because there are some players who could join together and bring a class-action suit against the NFL.

Harry Carson, 53, NFL Hall of Famer

I first learned about the NFL's concussion experts while I was watching television one day in November 2003. It was five months after my last wrestling match, and I had just started paying attention to the media's coverage of concussions. A friend told me that the HBO show *Inside the NFL* was going to air a feature on the research of the Center for the Study of Retired Athletes (CSRA), specifically on the link it has found between multiple concussions on the football field and an increased risk of depression.

Inside the NFL introduced the Center's findings, and then showed the NFL's reaction. The NFL spokesperson was Dr. Elliott Pellman, the New York Jets team doctor who also serves as chairman of the NFL Subcommittee on Mild Traumatic Brain Injury. I was eager to hear his thoughts on these provocative, but not unexpected, findings. To this day, I'm still shocked by his official response to the research.

"When I look at that study, I don't believe it,"[3] Pellman said.

I did a double-take. "I don't believe it" was not the reaction I'd expected from a man of science. Pellman was strangely defensive and dismissive. I figured that he could disagree with the study's findings in two ways: he could either find fault with the methodology (how the CSRA had conducted the study) or the conclusions (what the CSRA had inferred from the data). Instead, he took a rare third path—personal experience and anecdotal evidence.

> I don't believe those numbers. I have not seen that depression, that melancholy, that was described in that study.[4]

I saw the show months before I read any research on the short- and long-term associations between depression and concussions, so I didn't immediately realize how unlikely it was for Dr. Pellman to be so unfamiliar with depression in concussed football players. I thought to myself, "Pellman must know that just because he hasn't seen that depression himself doesn't mean that it doesn't exist." (I've never seen a germ, but I still wash my hands.) Besides, what are the odds that an NFL team doctor has the time to treat a large group of retired athletes, which is the subject of this research?

I became more disillusioned with the NFL's top concussion expert when he went on to offer an alternative explanation for why ex-NFL football players would be suffering from depression at such a high rate.

> You take any professional, and give them a window of opportunity of which 4, 5, 6, 7, 8 years is the pinnacle of their career, of which they've done what they've loved, what has consumed them, and now push them into an entirely different profession . . . what type of effect would that have on you?[5]

That statement sounds believable. However, a trained scientist would know that it cannot account for the findings of the study. All 2,500 people interviewed were ex-NFL players. The fact that they were all ex-NFL players is what is referred to in academia as a "controlled variable." If the study compared ex-NFL players to the general population, Pellman's "theory" could be true. But as the study was conducted, his theory would never explain why some ex-players are more prone to depression than others. It would require a variable that wasn't the same for every player, like the number of concussions in their lifetime, to account for the increased risk of depression.

Pellman continued to confuse me. He said,

> If we take a look at the tools we have now, there is no one else who
> is finding that element.[6]

Pellman was trying to isolate the study as an aberration, yet, as Dr. Omalu says, this study did not "come out of the deep blue sea." Research linking depression and traumatic brain injury has existed for years. It's easily discovered by searching for the term "depression" with either "concussion" or "traumatic brain injury" or "head injury" at the National Library of Medicine's medical journal search engine at http://www.ncbi.nlm.nih.gov/PubMed.[7] [8] [9] (Or if you prefer the search engine Google, you can type "head injury depression" at scholar.google.com and read the bevy of studies for yourself.)

In fact, Pellman's claim was so dubious that even *Inside the NFL,* which has a working relationship with the NFL and probably doesn't want to rock that boat, noted, "But *Inside the NFL* did find several studies, published in prestigious journals and dating as far back as 1994, that do indeed suggest a connection."

All in all, I found the show very disturbing.

▼▼▼

The NFL's subcommittee on mild traumatic brain injury was formed in 1994 by Commissioner Paul Tagliabue. Dr. Elliott Pellman was chosen to chair the committee because of his experience treating former Jets receiver Al Toon, the first active player to retire due to what we now call "post-concussion syndrome." Pellman described how he came to his position, "From the beginning of his professional career, Mr. Toon began to incur what we now recognize as concussions. . . . Unrecognized by everyone, including myself, these concussions began to worsen in the later years of his career. . . . On the basis of my experience with Mr. Toon, I was invited to the Commissioner's office to offer my limited insight into this problem. The Commissioner and I realized that we had many more questions than answers. . . . I was asked to mount an effort to answer these questions."[10]

The committee includes a neurosurgeon, a neurologist, a neuropsychologist, a biomechanical engineer, and an epidemiologist, but curiously is headed by Pellman, who is trained as an "internist and rheumatologist."[11]

When Dr. Omalu was forced to defend his work against the NFL concussion committee's attack, he shared my surprise, telling me, "When I learned that Pellman was a rheumatologist, I was amazed. The NFL didn't even include a neuropathologist on its committee."[12]

Two years after it formed the committee, the NFL began a five-year study on concussions in the NFL. The finding weren't released until 2003. Some believe that super-agent Leigh Steinberg—the man on whom Tom Cruise's *Jerry McGuire* character is based—helped motivate the NFL to conduct these studies by creating public pressure. Steinberg represented more than 100 players in the mid to late 1990s, including Troy Aikman and Steve Young. He told me that when his players began having concussion problems, "we started pushing the NFL for changes. First of all, if we can send a space probe to Mars, we ought to have the technology to create a helmet that can better protect the head. So I pushed for technology. Then we pushed for a neurologist to be on the sidelines and grade concussions. This meant that when a player came off the field, a neurologist would determine whether he had a '0.2,' '0.6,' etc. A higher score would mean that the player would have to sit out the game for a longer period of time. A play, a game, a week, two weeks—this period of rest would be standardized throughout the NFL. Then we pushed for the strict enforcement of a rule that the head and neck were not to be used in tackling—no spearing, no going for the head."

But the NFL wasn't receptive to Steinberg's ideas. He remembers, "The more I pushed for these things, the more blowback there was. At times it came from my own players, at times it came from a doctor like Elliot Pellman. I forget the exact quote, but Pellman said something to *Sports Illustrated* to the effect that I was a 'scaremonger'—and that the problems weren't as bad as I was making them out to be. Well, Pellman is not going to know Troy Aikman or Steve Young or Warren Moon or Drew Bledsoe when they are 50, and I will." Some of Steinberg's most important recommendations, including that a neurologist be on the sideline and that there be more standardized guidelines in treating concussions, have been repeated by former players.

Merril Hoge, who believes he was forced to retire partially because of the inadequate medical care he received following a concussion, is a big believer in standardized treatment. "I still wish that in order to avoid all the pressures of the game, there were a guideline implemented in the NFL for when a guy has experienced a certain kind of concussion. For example, if his symptoms are A, B, and C, then he has to sit for a week, or two weeks, etc. That would really take the pressure off the medical staff, the player, and the team. Teams pay players a lot of money to play, but the teams still have to treat them as human beings, not as numbers. I think sometimes that gets lost."

Any type of standard has yet to be implemented in the NFL. This has led to some curious, controversial, and even comical sideline concussion management in the NFL.

In October 2004, Brett Favre suffered a concussion in a game against the New York Giants. Favre was slammed to the ground by defensive lineman William Joseph. Packers coach Mike Sherman said Favre was a "little cloudy" after the hit, and the medical staff asked that he be taken out of the game.[13] Backup Doug Pedersen went in for the next two plays. On the sideline, Coach Sherman then asked Favre if he felt okay.

Favre, as most competitive athletes would, said yes. Sherman, without consulting with the team doctor or trainer, put Favre back in, where he immediately threw a 28-yard touchdown pass. Sherman said, "The doctors later told me that they didn't want to put him back in the game. The doctors hadn't exactly cleared him. So I was in error putting him back in the game." Giants quarterback Kurt Warner spoke with Favre as he came off the field and reported that Favre didn't remember the touchdown.

Kurt Warner was a victim of the same lack of communication just a year earlier. While playing for the St. Louis Rams, Warner suffered a concussion in the first half of a game against the New York Giants. The team doctor, Bernard T. Garfinkel, cleared him at halftime to return to play. In the second half, Warner was having trouble deciphering the plays. Clearly, he hadn't recovered. When Dr. Garfinkel was asked by the press why Warner had been allowed to continue to play in the second half even though he still appeared to be suffering from the effects of the concussion, the doctor said, "That's a coaching decision, not a medical decision."[14] If you notice, that hierarchy is the polar opposite of what Green Bay Packers Coach Mike Sherman had said about the Brett Favre incident. Apparently whether a doctor or coach has the final say over medical decisions varies by team.

Sometimes a player is told that he didn't have a concussion even though he's convinced that he did. After a game against the Cleveland Browns, Cincinnati Bengals wide receiver Chad Johnson told the press that he had suffered a mild concussion and didn't remember much after being tackled on a reception, including a 46-yard touchdown catch he'd made in the first quarter.[15] Yet Head Coach Marvin Lewis told the press that if Johnson had actually suffered a concussion of any sort, he wouldn't have been allowed to continue playing.

"I can say 100 percent, unequivocally that our medical staff wouldn't have allowed it," said Lewis. "[Wide receivers coach] Hue Jackson did say at a point that for a while after the touchdown catch, Chad wasn't feeling quite right, so they took him out for a few plays. But he cleared up, went back into the game, and was fine. It's fun and cool to be injured like the other guys once in a while." [16] So Johnson got tackled, didn't feel well, and the trainers thought enough of it to pull him from the game. But the coach says he didn't have a concussion. Who would you believe? The player or the coach?

Some coaches even have trouble understanding the definition of a concussion. After one game, Pittsburgh Steelers Head Coach Bill Cowher was asked by the press whether Duce Staley had suffered a concussion. He answered, "No, he was just a little groggy." [17] He was asked, "Did Ben Roethlisberger get knocked woozy?" He answered, "Yes . . . I think on the one point after his scramble . . . [But] there is no concussion." According the NFL's concussion definition, Cowher was 0 for 2 on those diagnoses.

Sometimes players convince officials to let them stay in after they've obviously suffered a concussion. In 2005, Dallas Cowboys offensive lineman Rob Petitti was kneed in the side of the head in a game. He got up woozy and unsteady on his feet. According to one journalist, the official noticed the injury, but Petitti convinced him to let him stay in, and the Dallas sideline did nothing. Before the next play, Cowboys quarterback Drew Bledsoe called timeout. Petitti could barely stand. When the timeout was over, Petitti stayed in the game. [18]

Sometimes the public relations department and the coaches end up on different pages. In 2004 San Diego Chargers center Nick Hardwick sustained a concussion in the first quarter of a game against the Raiders. The team announced that Hardwick would not return for the rest of the game. In the third quarter, he was back in the lineup. "I was out of it for a little while," said Hardwick, whose head began to clear in the middle of the second quarter. "I didn't know what was going on. I didn't know any plays. I didn't know what was what." [19]

The San Diego Chargers sideline was also the setting of one of the better-documented cases of confusing concussion treatment. In 2004 Drew Brees sustained a concussion during a Chargers-Jets game after taking a helmet-to-helmet hit from Jon McGraw. One play later, after a LaDainian Tomlinson touchdown, Brees went to the sideline, where the trainers asked him some standard concussion questions. "A couple of them I thought I answered OK, and the others maybe not," Brees said.[20] The trainers cleared him to go back in.

Offensive coordinator Cam Cameron asked Brees how he was feeling. "I guess I told him 60 percent," Brees said. "I just arbitrarily threw out a number. They saw me stumbling around on the sideline trying to pick up a ball to get loose again before I went back out."[21] Drew did go back out. In the huddle, Tomlinson noticed that Brees wasn't himself. Brees threw a touchdown pass and returned to the sideline. Coach Cameron told head coach Marty Schottenheimer about his conversation with Brees. The head coach had yet to be informed about the concussion. Without consulting team physicians, Schottenheimer immediately decided that Brees was done for the day.

Backup quarterback Doug Flutie remembered, "Drew didn't want to give up his spot. Not only did he have me as a backup, but the team had drafted Philip Rivers in the off-season. So when Brees got hit, and we all knew he was a little off, I picked up a ball and started warming up. But Brees went back in there and played really well, even throwing a great touchdown pass. So I put the ball down and stopped warming up. Then out of nowhere the offensive coordinator came over and said, 'You're going in.' I said, 'Are you serious?' I guess the doctors had been trying to evaluate Brees every time he came to the sideline during those 11 or so plays, but he just kept telling them he was fine."

I guess those doctors didn't have the authority to hold Drew out for a series to fully evaluate his condition.

That decision was covered in the San Diego sports pages that week; some sportswriters supported Schottenheimer for being concerned about Brees's well-being, while others admonished him for playing doctor. But the fact is that Brees was allowed to continue for eleven or twelve more plays while still symptomatic from an obvious concussion—precisely the kind of dangerous situation that Leigh Steinberg and Merril Hoge have been warning the NFL about for a decade.

Two of the best-known sports concussion treatment guidelines, written by the American Academy of Neurology and Dr. Robert Cantu, both recommend that any player with a concussion be monitored for at least fifteen minutes after a mild concussion, because symptoms can sometimes get worse or may not appear for a few minutes. The guidelines were created to protect a player from the consequences of secondary impacts, and because a concussed player is less able to protect himself from injury on the field. Even Elliott Pellman has published a paper discussing how some NFL players' symptoms are worse the day after the injury than the day of the injury, suggesting "that the mTBI sets off intracranial processes that result in worsening cognitive functioning over the first twenty-four to forty-eight hours after the injury."[22] Brees is the poster boy for fifteen minutes of rest, as Schottenheimer told reporters after the game, "I think it was something as he continued to play, it got worse."[23]

When Brees's teammate LaDainian Tomlinson was informed that the team expected Brees to play the next week, he said, "I don't think he should [play]. We're talking about someone's life here . . . For the safety of him, he shouldn't be out there. This could really affect him in the long run. In the short term, it isn't important for him to be playing with a concussion."[24] Tomlinson got it.

Others don't. These examples pale in comparison to the sideline care that the NFL's concussion guru, Dr. Elliott Pellman, gave to Wayne Chrebet, the latest NFL player to retire prematurely from multiple concussions. Understanding NFL concussion care can be difficult because doctors are rarely allowed to explain their sideline decisions to the media. Dr. Elliott Pellman is not one of those doctors. His explanations to the New York media revealed a great deal about his unique opinions on concussions.

The Curious Case of Wayne Chrebet

On November 2, 2003, New York Jets wide receiver Wayne Chrebet suffered a concussion in a game against the New York Giants. By all accounts, he lost consciousness for about a minute.[25] [26] [27] [28] Photographs show that Chrebet was still lying facedown on the turf when three members of the Jets medical staff reached him.[29]

A number of return-to-play guidelines for concussions exist so that medical personnel will know when it's safe for a player to return to the field. Each guideline varies slightly, but they all consistently say that if an athlete is knocked out for any length of time, he shouldn't return to the game. If Pellman had been following the Cantu guidelines, he would have advised holding Wayne Chrebet out for at least two weeks. If Pellman were using the AAN system, he would have rushed Chrebet to the hospital for overnight observation and kept him out of action for at least a week.

But Dr. Pellman cleared Chrebet to go back into the game. It would be the last game Chrebet played that season. All concussion guidelines leave room for clinical judgment, meaning that a doctor always has the right to overrule the guidelines. However, when the New York media forced Pellman to justify his decision to return Chrebet to action, he didn't use clinical judgment as his defense. Instead, Pellman applied some rather bizarre logic.

Three days after the game, Pellman was asked whether Chrebet was suffering post-concussion syndrome. He answered, "I don't know if Wayne is post-concussed or not. The fact that I don't know is why I'm a little nervous."[30] It isn't easy to say whether Wayne was suffering from post-concussion syndrome, as there is no true clinical definition. But Wayne was certainly suffering from post-concussion symptoms, as "Chrebet complained [to Pellman] of fatigue and some headache-like pain Monday night and early Wednesday [the two had no contact Tuesday]."[31]

Ten days after the game, Chrebet was placed on injured reserve (IR) for the season. The New York media began asking Pellman more pointed questions. It was obvious to everyone that when Chrebet returned to play in the Giants game, he had either not recovered from his concussion, or he had been exposed to secondary trauma, making the injury much worse. Or both.

Dr. Pellman defended his actions by saying, "The decision about Wayne returning to play was based on scientific evaluation and medical evaluation. That evaluation and that decision made no difference as to what's happening today."[32] He added, "Let's say I didn't allow him to return to play, and he played the following weekend. The same thing could have happened. I can only go by what we find scientifically."[33]

I'm not sure if the medical evidence supports those statements. Most, if not all, brain trauma experts agree that there is a period of vulnerability after a concussion occurs, where further trauma can cause greater injury or even death. (See Chapter 4.) Had he rested for a week, Chrebet would have had seven days to flush out the potassium and calcium that had collected in the wrong places in his brain while restoring normal cerebral blood flow.[34]

To add insult to secondary injury, Pellman told the press, "This will not be something that I will be concerned about for months, but it's been more than just a few days. There was no concern on any of our parts that Wayne will have any long-term problems."[35]

Perhaps the strangest exchange happened only moments before Chrebet went back into the game. According to Pellman, he'd told Chrebet, "This is very important. You can't lie to me. There's going to be some controversy about going back to play. This is very important for you, and this is very important for your career. Are you okay?" Chrebet reportedly answered, "I'm fine."[36][37]

Logic tells us that a man with a malfunctioning brain and without medical training would be a terrible judge of whether or not he should go back into the game. Logic tells us that a brain-damaged player with a large personal and financial incentive to lie to get back in the game is not the best person to ask. But perhaps Pellman simply isn't aware of that logic, nor of the concussion guidelines that urge doctors never to ask players if they "are okay."

I believe that Pellman is aware of the research. Among the dozens of papers I'd gotten from the library was an article titled "Concussion in Sports," published in *The American Journal of Sports Medicine*. The paper came out of a December 1997 concussion workshop sponsored by the American Orthopaedic Society of Sports Medicine in Chicago.[38] Most of the top sports concussion doctors were at this workshop, including my old Harvard team doctor, Art Boland, and Elliott Pellman.

If you assume that the concepts published in that study were discussed at the workshop, then Pellman should have been familiar with the idea that players aren't reliable. On page 681 of "Concussion in Sports," the authors wrote, "Many players will deny symptoms to be able to return to competition." They repeated the statement three pages later, writing, "It cannot be assumed that an athlete is normal when he or she 'feels fine.'" Even Leigh Steinberg thought that it was important enough to mention to me, saying, "There are so many problems with this area. One of them is that doctors ask players to evaluate their health when they are concussed."

When Chrebet was placed on injured reserve for the remainder of the season, a reporter asked Pellman if Chrebet would be at greater risk for future concussions and post-concussion problems. Pellman answered, "Is Wayne more susceptible now to these injuries? I do not know. But one of the things I believe is to try and prevent that susceptibility [by giving] the person a chance to recover."[39] By this I guess Pellman means that NFL players should have a chance to recover when the game is officially over, but not during the game.

Somehow Pellman was pulling off an amazing balancing act. A week earlier Pellman had said that he didn't second-guess sending Chrebet back into the game, implying that Chrebet wasn't at further risk.[40] Then a week later, he said that rest lowers the risk of further injury. He seemed to be creating some alternative medical universe where Chrebet wasn't at risk for further injury immediately after the concussion, but was suddenly at risk ten days later. Again, let me say that this same doctor published a paper suggesting "that the mTBI sets off intracranial processes that result in worsening cognitive functioning over the first twenty-four to forty-eight hours after the injury."[41] But I guess this just didn't hold true for Wayne Chrebet.

In reality, the risk of further injury immediately after getting knocked unconscious is so great that the "Concussion in Sports" workshop paper mentioned it four times on a single page.[42]

- The medical personnel at the competition may allow the athlete to return to play if there was no loss of consciousness and all signs and symptoms are normal.
- Any observed period of unconsciousness is significant and should always preclude return to play.
- Return to Play Classifications
  - Delayed Return to Play (Not the Same Day)
    - Documented loss of consciousness
- Recommendations
  - Loss of consciousness precludes return to play that day

Now I understand why Pellman said that he'd told Chrebet on the sideline, "There's going to be some controversy about going back to play." To me, it sounds like Pellman was sending a lamb to the slaughter, and, to cover himself, he pawned off the responsibility for his actions onto the lamb.

Chrebet's story does not have a happy ending. The injury that he received in the Giants game was his fifth recorded concussion since his freshman year of college—but may have been his sixth or seventh.[43] More than a month after the injury, Wayne said, "It just feels horrible, feels like people say you fell into a black hole. You wait to come out again. It's a crazy thing. Every morning you wake up feeling hung over, like you had the worst night of your life."[44]

In the off-season, the Jets renegotiated Chrebet's contract to include a concussion clause.[45] [46] Normally, if Chrebet were to end up on injured reserve, he'd be paid his full base salary of $1.5 million. The Jets added an unprecedented clause in his contract stating that if he ended up on IR from a concussion, he would earn only $500,000. In essence, the Jets gave Chrebet—the kind of guy who would get knocked unconscious and beg to go back in—increased financial incentive to hide any concussions from the team the next season.

Chrebet's 2004 season ended with another concussion; he received this one during the last game of the regular season. He sat out the Jets playoff game. His career finally came to an end when he suffered a concussion against the San Diego Chargers on November 6, 2005. His teammates were reportedly shaken by the sight of Chrebet as he lay unconscious on the field, his legs frozen in the air, and again in the locker room as trainer David Price had to help him undress. Chrebet was placed on the IR.[47] He was still suffering from symptoms daily when he officially retired on June 2, 2006, saying, "You wake up every morning like you have a hangover. I don't know why that is. I've been told it goes away eventually. I look forward to that day. You deal with a lot of inner demons and mixed emotions when you go through something like this. I go through a lot of days where I struggle. I'm not the same as I was years ago, let's put it that way. I wouldn't say you get used to it. You learn to expect it."[48]

From these examples and others, Dr. Elliott Pellman and the NFL team doctors seem radically out of step with the research and recommendations of the rest of medical community. Being a team doctor is a prestigious position, so the explanation could legitimately be that the NFL doctors are more qualified than their counterparts. But since many teams no longer choose their team doctors, there may be no correlation between being a team doctor and being a good doctor. A recent *New York Times* article exposed the current trend of doctors paying teams for the "right" to treat players because the promotional advantage is so lucrative.[49]

With doctors paying teams, the reason for their aggressive treatment of concussions may be much simpler. Dr. Delaney explains, "At the pro level, if you practiced the most conservative guidelines, you probably wouldn't be a pro doc very long. And that's the sad truth." Many doctors believe that paying teams creates a direct conflict of interest, as the doctors might be tempted to protect the team's interests rather than the players' in order to maintain their position.[50]

But Pellman's achievement of such a prestigious position might be the most interesting tale. As I've explained, some were surprised when the NFL appointed Pellman, who is not a neurologist, to head up its concussion committee. Pellman is no stranger to such controversy; he briefly became a household name in March 2005 for a string of missteps.

Pellman had been hired by Major League Baseball (MLB) as a medical advisor, and he defended its steroid policy before Congress in 2005. After giving a very pro-MLB opening statement, Pellman was hammered by several members of Congress on his lack of knowledge about MLB's steroid policies. It turns out that Pellman didn't know that players were allowed to leave the room for an hour in the middle of a drug test, and that they could be fined rather than suspended for positive tests.[51]

Representative Tom Lantos, a Democrat from California, called Pellman "pathetically unpersuasive," and said that he sounded like a tobacco industry official. Lantos also pointed out that Pellman's testimony undermined the contributions of the rest of the medical panel.[52][53] Representative Henry Waxman, another Democrat from California, said, "Major League Baseball told us Dr. Pellman was their foremost expert, but he was unable to answer even basic questions about the league's steroid policy at the hearing."[54]

This is the same Elliott Pellman who'd said in 2002 (before he was hired by MLB), "The players and the team owners have sold their souls to the devil with steroids, and I know, because I've been treating professional athletes since 1986."[55] That is quite an about-face.

Days after the hearing, the *New York Times* broke the story that Pellman had falsified his résumé.[56] Among four inaccuracies, Pellman claimed to have a medical degree from the State University of New York at Stony Brook. The truth is that Pellman graduated from the Universidad Autonoma de Guadalajara, in Mexico, and received a certificate of completion from SUNY Stony Brook. He was later awarded an MD degree by the State Department of Education.

Mexican medical schools have lower admissions standards than U.S. medical schools do. According to the *New York Times*, Dr. Pellman said that he had enrolled there in 1975 because of poor grades as a biology major at New York University. Dan Brock, director of Harvard Medical School's

Division of Medical Ethics, said, "If I told you I graduated from medical school in the United States, and I went to Guadalajara, then I think I would have deliberately misled you, so I would say that was unethical." [57]

If the NFL is wrong about its treatment of concussions, this could cause a serious problem for youth football. Many experts realize that NFL concussion management guidelines are followed at the lower levels of the game. Dr. Julian Bailes, a former neurosurgeon for the Pittsburgh Steelers, said, "We have cautioned against using the NFL management criteria and their way of thinking at the lower levels of play, because it's natural for people to want to emulate them. The NFL is not recommending its management practices; it's just saying 'that's how we do it.' The NFL is going to be emulated in everything it does. That's why it has such a huge responsibility. Whether it wants to admit it or not, it's an organizational role model."

Dr. Heechin Chae expresses similar concerns, saying, "Trainers or physicians at the college or high-school level need some kind of example to follow. So if the NFL has different standards, they're going to follow that standard too."

Others believe that the concern lies less with the youth trainers who follow the lead of the NFL, and more with the young players who try to emulate their NFL role models. After watching Brett Favre suffer a concussion, and then go back into the game to throw a touchdown, one Wisconsin prep football player remarked, "I kind of wonder how they can do it yet we can't do it, but it was amazing how he went right back in and threw a touchdown." [58]

▼▼▼

The NFL's unique perspective on concussions goes beyond treatment and interpretation of other groups' research. The NFL got into the concussion research business itself in 1996, and its 5-year study has been released in 11 articles (thus far) series in the medical journal *Neurosurgery*, with Pellman listed as the primary author. The papers have caused a controversy in the medical community. As one prominent researcher (who asked not to be named due to a business affiliation with the NFL) told me, "Where it's challenging for someone like me is how the NFL is extrapolating their research to the entire population, and how they say they don't have a head injury problem, because they clearly do. The fact is those papers are becoming everyone's gospel, and that's dangerous."

The most controversial paper is Part Four, regarding players who sustained more than one concussion. Pellman says that their research did not find a higher risk of repeated concussions in players with previous concussions, and that there was no "7- to 10-day window of increased susceptibility to sustaining another concussion."[59]

Neurosurgery is a "peer-reviewed" journal, meaning that every article is sent to prominent doctors for their comments before it's published, and then the study and the comments are published together. Dr. Bailes explains, "Editorial comments provide the reader, most of the time a physician, another point of view or context from other experts in the same field." Dr. Cantu was one of the article's reviewers, and noted: "At first glance, the NFL experience with single and repeat concussion (no difference) and management (more than 50 percent of players return to the same game, including more than 25 percent of those with loss of consciousness) seems to be at odds with virtually all published guidelines and consensus statements on managing concussion."

Another doctor wrote, "Unfortunately, the present article in this series of studies on professional football players has several flaws with respect to the study design, data collection, and data analyses. . . . The article sends a message that it is acceptable to return players while still symptomatic, which contradicts literature published over the past twenty years suggesting that athletes be returned to play only after they are asymptomatic, and in some cases for seven days." He goes on to point out, rightly, that the studies the NFL tries to discredit have collected more data more often, using more sophisticated tests, including computerized neuropsychological screenings. The NFL data was based solely on clinical analysis, verbal questions, and pencil-and-paper tests, which are either less sensitive and/or more subjective than the methods the NFL group chooses to bash.

Part Six, which deals with neuropsychological testing and concluded, "there is no evidence in this study of widespread permanent or cumulative effects of single or multiple mTBI's in professional football players," was also blasted by the peer reviewers.[60] The first reviewer called the conclusions "premature." The second said the results should be interpreted with "caution," especially considering that 78 percent of concussed players chose not to take the neuropsychological tests. That means four out of five players refused to be tested. Why would an athlete refuse the test? My guess is that it's for the same reason that people pulled over on suspicion of driving drunk refuse a breathalyzer test . . . because they don't want anyone to have proof that they were compromised.

The third reviewer called the methodological choices "perplexing." The fifth reviewer pointed out the same flaws the others had, while expressing exasperation that Pellman drew the conclusions he did considering that the NFL study only looked at short-term symptoms, and by virtue of the study design, it didn't follow players who had retired from the cumulative effects of concussion. (You won't find cancer in a study population if you take out the people who have it!)

Even the fourth reviewer, Dr. Joseph Maroon, the Steelers neurosurgeon who usually plays the role of NFL cheerleader in these peer review sections, wrote, "It is specifically recommended that the statement that there are no widespread permanent or cumulative effects of single or multiple mTBIs in professional football players be softened somewhat."

This strong backlash from their peers makes me wonder why the NFL doctors were trying so hard to make the case that multiple concussions are no worse than a single concussion, and that there are no negative long-term consequences from concussions. I can't come up with an answer. Maybe, as NFL Hall of Famer Harry Carson told me, they're worried about lawsuits from players.

But let's say that the NFL doctors are correct. Let's say that, because the NFL players are older, they're not exposed to the risks younger players are. If that were true, then we would have to find another way to spread the word about the risks of concussion to younger players, because the NFL is certainly not going to play that role. The *Christian Science Monitor* reported, "In its TV ads, the National Football League emphasizes the hard hits, the quarterback sacks, and the razor-edged intensity of the professional game. But when it comes to youth sports, the NFL is calling for a tamer approach, one that de-emphasizes violence and competition and emphasizes safety, fun, and teamwork."[61] Scott Lancaster, the director of NFL Youth Development, says that it has a three-pronged plan to "take out all the negatives and emphasize the positives."[62] The NFL has run over four million children through its numerous youth programs, which include Junior Player Development, High School Player Development, Pass, Punt, and Kick, USA Football, and NFL Canada. It has also developed quite a presence on the Internet. Its sites include www.playfootball.com, "The Official NFL Website for Kids"; www.NFLCFLFutures.com, a partnership between NFL and CFL to promote youth football; www.nflhs.com, the NFL's Official Site for High School Football; www.usafootball.com, founded by the NFL to promote youth participation in football; and www.nflcanada.com, founded by the NFL to promote football in Canada.[63]

Scott Lancaster gave a seminar at a conference on marketing to children in 2005 that was called, "Making Your Brand Kid-Cool and Mom Acceptable." According to Leigh de Armas, a journalist who attended the conference, Lancaster said that children are important to the NFL because getting the attention of a kid means better odds of creating an adult football fan with some discretionary income.[64]

But Lancaster knows that the NFL can't get to kids without going through moms. "It's important to create a product that moms will embrace," he reportedly said. "One of the most radical things we did with our football clinics is we made soccer moms the coaches of tackle football. A lot of times you'll hear a kid say he can't play football because his parents don't approve, or they don't want him to get hurt. By bringing the mother in to coach, we were not only empowering the mothers, we were appealing to the fact that when children reach the ages of between 12 and 14, mothers will want to spend more time with their kids. This is the age when a lot of kids start slipping away to do their own thing. So by involving the mom, we were not only getting parent participation, it's great exposure for the brand."[65]

By itself, the NFL's marketing message to children isn't that bad. Many companies use similar tactics. But something changes when you combine a marketing program aimed at children and parents that is meant to "take out all the negatives and emphasize the positives" with a top doctor's radical statements such as, "If there's normal testing and a player feels good, what's the contraindication to letting him play? There really is none."[66] Based on its past behavior, I think we can be confident that the NFL is not going to sound any alarms about concussions in children. As Dr. Art Day, director of the Neurological Sports Injury Center at Brigham and Women's Hospital in Boston, says, "You're asking the fox if there's a particular problem with hanging around the henhouse. Pellman works for the NFL. Until there's definitive evidence otherwise, he's going to take that tack that managing concussions isn't a problem. Will Mercedes tell you they're not the best car?" [67]

▼▼▼

As concerned as I am for NFL players, they still have better access to medical care than players at any other level of the game. While NFL players can see trainers, doctors, neurologists, neurosurgeons and neuropyschiatrists relatively easily, a high-school, junior-high, or youth league football player does not have that luxury. In fact, only 30 to 33 percent of all high-schools have a certified athletic trainer on staff, and the trainer's time is divided among multiple sports.[68] So it's up to coaches, parents, and players to change how we approach concussions in football. That begins with a thorough understanding of how to prevent, diagnose, and treat them. And a sound discussion of concussion prevention begins by looking at football helmets.

CHAPTER 9

The Causes of the Concussion Epidemic

Football players are getting bigger, faster, and stronger, and they're wearing lighter and lighter equipment. When do we start building them too big and too fast? What happens when you don't have anyone left to play the games?

Mike Goforth, Virginia Tech head athletic trainer[1]

The impact to the head is the thing you cannot see if you haven't played.

Frank Rochon, 32, former high-school football player

Concussions have always been—and will always be—a part of the game. Regardless of how advanced the equipment is, because of the nature of the game, you're going to have concussions. When you're moving at a high rate of speed and you're forced to stop, your brain continues to move. If it hits up against the inside of your skull, it's going to put a bruise on your brain.

Harry Carson, 53, NFL Hall of Famer

Reducing both concussions and their negative consequences is a daunting task. The simplest way to solve football's concussion crisis is to prevent concussions from happening at all. The public discussion on prevention focuses on new football helmets, so when I speak with parents and players about prevention, they always ask, "Don't the new helmets prevent concussions?" Before I began this project, I too thought that technology would save us. Yet now that I understand the causes of the concussion epidemic, my faith in helmets has been severely diminished. That's not the message that the football and helmet industries want you to hear. But to come to that conclusion, all you have to do is take a step back and look at the evolution of the game and its head protection—an evolution that has made helmet-to-helmet hits an accepted part of the game.

I had graduated before Ray Hill began his Harvard football career, but I recognized his name from hearing it over the Harvard Stadium public-address system on Saturday afternoons. Ray was a linebacker and special teams player—the kind of guy who was known for making big hits. But Ray considered himself an honest big hitter. "I've tried to avoid 'leading with the head,'" he said. "I've always been taught, 'Go in with your facemask and your neck bold. Don't go in head down.' The first contact is usually my facemask, ideally facemask on the numbers. With my best hits, I'd hear the other guy lose his breath. I'd hear a 'whoosh.'"

I'd tracked Ray down because I'd heard he was retiring before his senior season was over because of a concussion. A mutual friend had tipped me off to his situation, but all I knew was that "he had a hell of a concussion story." When I called, Ray offered to meet with me at his dorm. He was living in the "Quad," an isolated area of residential housing at Harvard that I'd visited only a half-dozen times as student. When I arrived, I felt jealous. I'd heard that Quad rooms were bigger than the rooms in the "River Houses" where I had lived, but I didn't anticipate walking into a room that was huge, sunny, *and* had a kitchen. (Lousy "quadlings.") Ray was still living with members of the team, but since they were all at practice, we had the place to ourselves. Ray shared his rather unfortunate series of events with me. Our mutual friend hadn't exaggerated.

"I was on kickoff," Ray began. "I was running down and saw a double team coming at me. I figured I had to break up the double team, so I started speeding up a little to take on the two guys. It turned out that the double team was a distraction, and the two guys broke and went after somebody else. To block me, they peeled a front line guy back. He came out of my blind side, and I went head-to-head with him with the same force that I was going to hit two guys with.

"He connected with the side of my skull, but he ended up taking the worst of it . . . he got knocked completely out. When I got hit, I saw this bright white flash, and I felt like I'd had the wind knocked out of me. I stayed in for the next few plays, not really able to breathe, and then I went to the sideline and took a knee to catch my breath. When I stood up, I kind of wobbled, and I thought, 'Oh man, this is not good.' But I didn't really think too much of it. I had a couple of plays to recover, and then I was back on the field for punt team. I played the rest of the game. After the game I only had a headache, but I told the trainers what had happened anyway. They told me that I had probably gotten a concussion, and to come back the next day and see them.

"That night, I hung out with my roommates—the doctors had told them to keep me awake for the next eight hours, just in case. As the night went on, I started getting really loopy, really 'out of it.' I went down to the convenience store for some sodas and stuff. I was standing in line for at least thirty seconds before I realized that the woman ahead of me in line was telling me to go ahead of her. I hadn't noticed that she was saying anything to me. I ended up going to bed at midnight, very early for a Saturday night, and I slept until one o'clock the next day, Sunday. That meant I was late for the noon training room check-in. When I woke up, I was still loopy, with no idea of what was going on. I hustled down to the trainers and said, 'I'm really messed up.'

"The doctors gave me a concussion test. At one point they tested my vision. They had me cover one eye and read some newsprint. When I covered my right eye, I could see fine. But when I covered my left eye, there was nothing. For the first time that day, I realized I couldn't see out of my right eye at all!

"They sent me to the hospital, where I had a CAT scan and an MRI. Both tests were negative. They made me stay at University Health Services hospital for a few days to recover. An ophthalmologist said there was a little bit of swelling of the optic nerve. That could cause some blurriness of both eyes, but not just one, so he was at a total loss. He didn't know what the problem could be.

"I ended up seeing four or five different doctors. They were all at a loss. One of the more prominent doctors theorized that the impact had triggered a muscle spasm in an arterial wall of an artery to my eye, basically cutting off blood flow and causing blindness. But they really had no idea; it was just a best guess. I've had a lot of injuries in general, so I'm used to tolerating them, but this was an adjustment. There were times that I thought that this would damage me for the rest of my life. The doctors said that they didn't see any reason why the problem shouldn't fix itself, and I had to take their word for it. It was scary.

"I couldn't see out of my right eye at all for about two weeks. I couldn't go to class, and even after that I had a real hard time reading or focusing. My depth perception was also doing some fun things. It gradually returned over the next couple of months.

"The post-concussion symptoms came in waves and lasted for a few months. There were times when I would feel really 'out of it,' especially if

I was trying to read; I couldn't look at a book for more than ten minutes before I started to space out. There were times when I'd get up fast and get a head rush; that obviously had happened before, but now it was happening a lot more often. I was also more lethargic, and had a lot less energy than usual. I slept a lot during the day. I couldn't stay awake. It was a tough time. Every once in a while I still experience some dizziness, and my vision gets a little shaky. I'm hoping that goes away completely in the next couple months.

"I've decided not to play during my senior year. The doctors have said, 'We can't really be sure, but we can't risk you going back and getting hit again. You could be susceptible to this kind of injury now. The problem could worsen, or it could come back more frequently.' So, that was pretty much the end of it."

Ray's injury was caused by a helmet-to-helmet hit. In the NFL, two out of every three concussions are caused by helmet-to-helmet hits—not by the helmet hitting the ground, other parts of the body, or by whiplash.[2] Logically, to reduce the incidence of concussions, we would have to reduce those caused by helmet-to-helmet hits, or simply reduce helmet-to-helmet hits altogether. Ray's situation was unique in that both players apparently suffered a concussion on the same play. This only happens in a tiny fraction of impacts: Studies show that in most situations, the concussion is caused by one player purposely driving his forehead into another player's helmet when that second player is relatively defenseless.[3] Previously I'd only thought of helmets in a positive light, such as, "Thank goodness that player had a helmet on, or he'd be dead." But I'd never thought, "If that player didn't have that helmet on, that head-to-head collision would have never happened." So, for a purely academic exercise, I turned the problem upside down. What if helmets aren't the solution to the concussion problem in football, but the cause?

That statement starts to make sense if we look at the evolution of helmets. After all, helmets weren't always part of the game. When Princeton and Rutgers played the first football game on November 6, 1869, the players wore nothing on their heads, and their football game was more like a game of rugby. The only protection the players had for their heads was their long hair.[4] While I wasn't there to watch that game, I can imagine from my experiences playing street football that head-to-head contact was probably avoided at all costs. But players still occasionally bashed skulls, and with dire consequences. This led Rutgers University to invent the leather football helmet in 1896.[5] Whatever the effect that leather helmets had on injuries, it wasn't enough, and the deaths and catastrophic injuries mounted.

The 1905 season left 18 players dead and 159 seriously injured, an astonishing total considering that there weren't nearly as many participants in the game as there are today.[6] President Theodore Roosevelt, in response to this tragic loss of life, threatened to ban the sport. His involvement led to the formation of the National Collegiate Athletic Association (NCAA), which was intended to be a rule-making body with the mandate to make participation in all college athletic programs safer.[7] At about this time, Harvard University President Charles Eliot led a movement to ban football at Harvard and at other colleges because he believed that football "incapacitated students for intellectual activity."[8] The game was banned at Northwestern, MIT, Columbia, Trinity, and Duke.[9]

In 1907, a task force was created to make the game of football safer. A group led by legendary Yale coach Walter Camp wanted to widen the field, which logically would reduce the frequency and intensity of player collisions.[10] But Harvard Stadium had just been built at a cost of $310,000.[11] Seating about 40,000 for football games, it was the largest reinforced concrete structure in the world. Unfortunately for the Walter Camp faction, the walls of Harvard Stadium couldn't be moved to widen the field, and far too much money had been put into its construction to render it obsolete. Instead, the forward pass was legalized. That, plus the narrow field, helped lead to the bone-jarring open-field hits that we see today.

In the early 1900s, the main causes of death from head injuries in football were due to skull fractures and bleeding on the brain. So, when the technology became available, someone created a stronger helmet surface to protect the brain. In 1917, the first hard-shelled, plastic helmet was introduced. This helmet didn't become standard until the NCAA mandated protective headgear in 1939.[12] These early helmets were suspended above the scalp by a webbing, and were successful in reducing serious injury. Dr. Cantu explained, "Helmets have reduced the instance of subdural hematomas [bleeding on the brain] by about 70 percent, the most life-threatening injury in football."

While the hard-shelled helmets were eventually preferred to their leather predecessors, they still didn't prevent facial injuries—especially to the eyes, mouth, and nose. Arguably, the biggest impact that the plastic helmet had on the way the game was played wasn't due to the helmet itself, but what could be attached to it. The hard plastic provided a solid anchoring point for plastic bars to be positioned across a player's face, allowing for the widespread adoption of the facemask. Over time, facemasks have evolved from one bar to two bars to today's grills, which allow players to lead with their faces with little fear of having an eye poked out or their teeth knocked in.

Surprisingly, while the hard-shelled helmet and facemask each made sense, the combination of the two proved deadly. Football deaths have been recorded since 1931. As the use of facemasks grew, and the facemask became more protective, catastrophic injuries swelled. They peaked in 1968, when thirty-six players died from football injuries and thirty men were permanently paralyzed.[13]

Football Head-Related Fatalities by Decade[14]

Years	Head Related Fatalities
1945–1954	87
1955–1964	115
1965–1974	162

Frederick Mueller, a leading authority on football-related head injuries, explained what happened. "The increase in fatal head injuries that began in the early 1960s and continued into the early 1970s can be directly related to the skills of tackling and blocking that were being taught during those years."[15] This period in football became known for tactics such as spearing, butt blocking, face to the numbers, and face in the chest. Players were being taught to make initial contact with the head and face into the opponent's chest.

The problem was partially one of design. The helmet was designed to protect the skull alone—there was little knowledge of the physics of concussions back then—and the helmet's effect on the brain was an afterthought. Merill Hoge captured this concept: "No helmet can eliminate trauma. To do that, you'd have to put a little helmet inside the skull, because the brain floats inside there. People need to understand that the helmet is there to protect the skull. It's not there to protect the brain, because that's impossible."

Facemasks removed the one thing that kept players from hitting each other with their head—fear. Fear of pain, fear of losing an eye. The head—once something to be protected—became something that could be used as a weapon to improve play. Anyone who watches old football games can see what a different role the head used to play. My "Aha!" moment came when I caught some clips of the famous 1968 Harvard-Yale game. Harvard scored

16 points in the final forty-two seconds, and "won" the game 29 to 29. As I watched the film, I was shocked to see that players purposely arm-tackled, ankle-tackled, and used other inefficient ways of getting an opponent to the ground.

Whitey Baun, the 54-year-old former college football player and current youth coach, gave some insight into that era. "When I started playing, they had just started changing the helmets, and the facemask would go right into the sternum," he told me. "You started really blasting people, and man, those hits were so sweet—like a drug. When I'm coaching kids now and I see those hits, it's an emotional high. It's like, 'Oh baby, that was it!' But maybe there's something wrong with those hits. Today we're teaching kids to run through other kids. I remember years ago when were taught to tackle. We would hit, roll, and take someone down to the ground. But now it's a collision—force to force."

To stem the tide of catastrophic injuries, a rule change was made in 1976 that prohibited initial contact with the head or face (contact known as spearing and butt blocking). According to some, this rule resulted in a dramatic decrease in both fatal head and cervical spine injuries.[16] It's true that direct fatalities from football have been reduced to the single digits each year since 1978. Yet some experts believe that the game is still marred by players' leading with their heads, making it not much safer than it was in the early 1970s. David Halstead, PhD, one of the leading experts on football helmets, has written that improved equipment and rules have probably made some small difference in reducing catastrophic injuries, but the real reason behind the decline "may be improved medical treatment."[17] Better emergency medicine combined with more advanced neurosurgery may help the more seriously injured athletes to survive.

Although this may seem like a big "maybe," consider the evidence. One study that analyzed footage of high-school football games found an average of forty head-down collisions per game involving just the ballcarrier in both 1975 and 1990.[18] [19] More than half of kickoffs lead to head-down collisions that involve the ballcarrier, making it the most dangerous play in football. (The kickoff team isn't called the "Suicide Squad" for nothing.) Depending on the study, head-down contact involving just the tacklers and ballcarriers occurs during between 6 and 26 percent of plays.

The NFL concussion study, despite its flaws, added to this body of evidence by re-creating concussion-causing impacts and other major hits using dummies in a laboratory. In every single instance, the study found that the striking player (usually the tackler or blocker) initiates contact with the crown of his own helmet, above his eyes and below the top of head.[20]

The head of the player who was struck experienced an average impact speed of 20.8 miles/hour, with a change in velocity of 16.1 miles/hour occurring over 15 milliseconds. In a car accident, the duration of a head injury is under 6 milliseconds if the head hits part of the structure of the car. A seatbelt and airbag will slow it down to about 40 milliseconds, meaning that the force is absorbed over a longer period of time, reaches a lower peak, and causes less damage. Football hits are closer to the former than the latter.[21] As a point of reference, if you drop a helmet from chest height (5 feet), it will hit the ground with an impact velocity of about 12 miles/hour.[22] To simulate those NFL hits, you'd have to drop the helmet from even higher—and you'd have to imagine your head inside of it.

Another way to measure the force is called "G's". One G is the force of gravity at sea level. The peak translational acceleration on the twenty-five recreated concussion-causing hits averaged 98 G's, with a range of 48–134 G's.[23] The rotational forces (not measured in G's) exceeded previously proposed life-threatening limits. A similar study was performed at Virginia Tech University (VT), but those researchers recorded hits from actual games. They found that half of all the hits measure greater than 30 G's, and the hardest hits are more than 130 G's. Stefan Duma, director of the Virginia Tech Center for Injury Biomechanics and an author of that study said, "An impact of 120 G's would be like a severe car accident, which you could survive if you were wearing a seat belt."[24] Mike Goforth, VT's head athletic trainer, said, "We were surprised. That's like running your head into a brick wall."[25]

You might think that the easiest way to eliminate these ferocious helmet-to-helmet impacts would be to change the rules and make these hits illegal. Amazingly, they already are illegal, and have been for years. Until 2005, the NCAA rule stated: "Intentional helmet-to-helmet contact is never legal, nor is any blow directed toward an opponent's head. Flagrant offenders should be disqualified."[26] High schools made butt blocking and face tackling illegal in 1976.

Considering how we remember playing the game, and how we watch it played today, many former players have a hard time believing in the integrity of those rules. Merril Hoge said, "You try to use your shoulder pads, but it's hard not to use your head. If you think your head's not going to get hit in some way, you're an absolute moron. When people are going at the speed they are going, you're going to get your head involved, and to deny that means you've never played the game."

In the NCAA, the concept of "intentional" helmet-to-helmet contact was so nebulous that it was virtually unenforceable. Spearing was not called as a penalty in 12 of the 20 major Division 1 conferences in 2001.[27] [28] In those major conference NCAA Division 1 games, 20,837 penalties were called, but only 17 were for spearing, and 8 for butting or ramming with the head. That equals one spearing penalty every 73 games, and one butting/ramming penalty every 156 games.

In 2005, the NCAA removed the word "intentional" from the rule to increase its enforcement and reduce helmet-to-helmet collisions. It worked, but not as the NCAA had hoped. Only 17 additional spearing and butting/ramming penalties were called in all of NCAA Division 1 football, an increase of less than one penalty per conference.[29]

My teammates and I used to sit around the locker room after games, comparing the new dents, scratches, and chips in our helmets and bragging about the collisions that had caused them. They were a badge of honor. Chipping the rubber off of the facemask to expose the metal was impressive, but actually bending a bar of the facemask was even better. I'd sit at my locker and run my fingers over the grooves on my helmet that were filled with paint from the opponent's helmets. By the end of the season, my helmet would look like a rainbow, with streaks of orange from Princeton, red from Cornell, and purple from Holy Cross.

This will give you an idea of what is considered legal: I once tackled a guy using only my facemask and wasn't flagged. It was my senior year. Princeton had a pretty good tailback, who was on the smallish side at about 170 pounds. I weighed in at 295 at that time. On one play, they tried to run the tailback up the gap between the opposite guard and center. I was getting blocked back by the center and (true to the Princeton tradition) he was cheating, holding my arm nearest to where the tailback was running. As the back was hitting the hole, I used the only thing available to hit him—my head. I head-butted him in the face as hard as I could, facemask-to-facemask, and somehow I knocked him flat on his back.

The scene on the field was kind of amusing. It had happened so quickly that my teammates didn't see the hit. Heck, I couldn't even be sure it was the running back whom I'd hit. We all stood in the huddle after the play, but no one congratulated each other. A teammate on the sideline told me that they were theorizing that the running back had been shot by a sniper. It all became clear at the film session the next day, when a coach made me out to be a hero for my resourcefulness on that play. We watched the play over and over in slow motion.

Because players are so well protected by their helmets and facemasks, preventing them from using their heads to tackle and block will be difficult. The NCAA experiment proved that enforcing the current rules that already make helmet-to-helmet hits illegal may be impossible. But if we can't prevent helmet-to-helmet contact, perhaps we can make it less harmful.

▼▼▼

Reducing the force that reaches the brain when helmets collide would lessen the concussion problem. Improvements have been made in the helmet's ability to absorb some of the impact before the energy reaches the brain. For example, in the 1990s, a study found that foam absorbs more force than suspension webbing in helmets, so manufacturers began changing what they put inside the shell.[30] But our ability to continue to improve these helmets is limited.

To understand why, we need to use a little physics. (I promise that it will be relatively painless.) Energy is neither created nor destroyed in a collision—it's transferred or absorbed. The problem with today's helmets is that too much energy is being transferred to and absorbed by the brain. One good way to prevent some of the force from reaching the brain in a collision is to use a single-use helmet. Single-use helmets, like bicycle and motorcycle helmets, are designed to be destroyed in a collision. This improves the outcome for the wearer in two ways. First, the foam on the inside of the helmet is designed to permanently deform, and second, the plastic is designed to crack. Both processes expend a large amount of energy that will thus not reach the brain. This is the same logic that is used in automobile crumple zones. The destruction of the body of the automobile absorbs some of the energy to protect the fragile person inside. The deforming foam also slightly prolongs the time that it takes for the brain to stop moving, lowering the peak force.

Unfortunately, a football helmet cannot be designed to crack, nor can the foam be designed to deform. A player often takes multiple hits to the helmet on a single play. If the helmet cracked or the foam were crushed after the first impact, the player would have no protection from other hits. Therefore, the primary responsibility of a football helmet is to not break. Merril Hoge knows this as well as anyone. He explained, "The helmets in the NFL are designed to withstand collisions. You look at NASCAR racers, and you'll see that their helmets are much better than the NFL helmets because they're designed to absorb contact and collisions and to minimize trauma." The design of a football helmet will always be limited by the nature of the game.

Now let's look at the helmet from another perspective—the helmet as a weapon. If the helmet is always going to be hard, any improvements that are made to it will be offset by the increased likelihood that the player will use the helmet more aggressively. If you have an ill-fitting helmet, it hurts when you hit someone, so you probably won't try to do that. But if it's painless, it's open season on leading with the head. There's no deterrent.

This phenomenon cuts across all sports, and is the main argument against soccer helmets. Helmet expert David Halstead, PhD, has written, "Parts of the body where equipment with improved impact protection is worn may be used more aggressively just as a result of having that area protected."[31] Another prominent researcher agrees, saying that children with better protective gear tend to take greater on-field risks, "paradoxically increasing their risk of sustaining a concussion injury by wearing a 'protective' helmet."[32] One study found that skiers and snowboarders who wear helmets travel 3mph faster down the slopes than people who don't.[33]

So with any improvement in helmets, we risk increasing the recklessness of the game. Interestingly, both offensive and defensive players have become equally unprotected. You might think that offensive players might be more prone to concussions because they're the ones who are getting tackled and sacked, but the NFL found that the concussion split between the tackler and tackled and between the blocker and the blockee was nearly 50/50.[34] What really matters is which player brings more force to the collision, and which player doesn't see the hit coming.

Since it's pretty well established that players are hitting each other in the head as hard as they can, I can say with confidence that helmets will never fix the problem. There are two forces involved in a hit to the head—linear and rotational. Linear forces knock the brain forward or backward in a straight line. Rotational forces twist the head, like a boxer taking a hook to the chin.

Helmets do a terrific job of preventing linear forces from reaching the brain, but they do a terrible job of limiting rotational forces. David Halstead has written, "Many of the remaining head injuries that occur on the field today may have rotational acceleration as the primary injury mechanism. Helmets would not prevent these injuries."[35] If we assume that rotational forces are the primary culprit for concussions, or even play a significant role, then we cannot prevent concussions. Dr. Halstead emphasized, "The helmet was not designed, and cannot be designed in the current state of the art . . . to prevent injuries to the brain which result from rotational acceleration." Halstead isn't the only expert to say this.[36] In his article "Birth and Evolution of the Football Helmet," published in the journal *Neurosurgery*, Michael Levy, MD, PhD, writes, "The American football helmet was and is designed to protect the areas of the player's head directly covered by the helmet from direct linear impact only. The helmet was not and cannot be designed to prevent . . . injuries to the brain that result from rotational acceleration."[37]

Taking this logic even further (and perhaps out onto a limb), if any improvement we make in helmets only serves to reduce linear forces (which is true), and that improvement makes players more likely to make contact with the head or allows them to deliver more punishing hits (also true), "improving" helmets could paradoxically increase the strength of the rotational forces that reach the brain, increasing the severity of rotational injuries, and possibly making the player less safe overall.

Increasing the potential for strong rotational forces in impacts is especially dangerous because research has shown that brain injuries caused by rotational forces tend to be more severe than those caused by linear forces. As Dr. Cantu explained, "Animal work was done by Ommaya and Gennarelli years ago.[38] They found that when they injured these animals by blows that were to the side of the head, the animals had more horrific injuries than they did by blows that were straight to the front, or straight to the back. They thought that was due to the fact that the brain stem was more likely angulated by those kinds of blows. So there is some animal work to suggest that if you take a shot to the ear, it may have a greater effect on you than a shot to the forehead would."

As it is well established that rotational forces have a major role in football concussions, and that football helmets do little to reduce those forces, we could skip the discussion of the benefits of the newest football helmets, the Riddell "Revolution" and the Schutt "DNA." If they make any difference it all, it would be minor. But overlooking these helmets wouldn't be any fun, because both these companies are spending a lot of money to get you to buy these newer and more expensive helmets. You deserve to know what's really going on.

Riddell and Schutt, the two biggest football helmet manufacturers, have recently introduced slick new helmets designs. Riddell says, "The Revolution is the first helmet using new technology, designed with the intent of reducing the risk of concussion."[39] Schutt says that the DNA was "designed with insights from an NFL-sponsored study of concussions."[40]

In discussing that research, the NFL's Dr. Pellman has said, "According to the scientists' research funded by the NFL, the current helmets underprotected the side of the head. The standard drop tests really didn't do any tests to the side of the head, so the [current] helmets were never really protected there. Riddell went to the scientists who did this research and integrated it into their own findings."[41] To understand exactly what he and Riddell are talking about, we need a little background on how helmets are tested and certified for use.

The "drop tests" that Pellman mentions are performed by the National Operating Committee on Standards for Athletic Equipment (NOCSAE), the governing body that certifies helmets. In a drop test, a football helmet is dropped from various heights to see how well it reduces the forces that reach the head at speeds up to 12 miles per hour. All NOCSAE tests involve linear forces—there are no tests or standards for rotational forces. (Naturally.)

The force is measured by a "severity index" (SI). The lower the number, the more protection a helmet provides. NOCSAE currently requires that new football helmets receive an SI score of 1200 or less on any test, because that level of protection has been found to effectively prevent most subdural hematomas. Dr. Cantu notes, "The brand new helmets that come right off the shelf are about 800, way better than the letter of the rule. Over the course of a season, or seasons, they get worse. But if you are going to protect against concussion, you are going to have to get down to a severity index of less than 300. Right now we're not even remotely close."

But the NOCSAE standard has no teeth, because there is no standard for the frequency of recertification or reconditioning of helmets.[42] Helmets become less effective the more they are used, so only the programs that have sufficient funding send helmets away every year to get fixed up, tested, and re-certified. This supposedly keeps older, ineffective helmets out of circulation. But it costs money to get helmets recertified, so in theory, a cash-strapped program could avoid having its broken-down, 20-year-old helmets declared to be illegal by never sending them for retesting. That's right: a worn-out hel-met remains certified and approved by NOCSAE as long as it isn't sent in for recertification testing. NOCSAE certification isn't proof that a helmet will pass certification on any given day, only that it once passed a certification test.

With that background, let's reexamine Pellman's statement. He claimed, "Current helmets underprotected the side of the head. The standard drop tests really didn't do any tests to the side of the head, so the [current] hel-mets were never really protected there." He bases his "underprotected" claim on the fact that many concussions in the NFL study were caused by players' getting hit in the side of the head. While that is an "interesting" conclusion to draw from those studies, it seems to ignore a crucial question that would lead to an entirely different (and less profitable) conclusion: Why would a football player get hit in the side of the head in the first place?

While I played, if I saw a helmet coming toward my head, I tried to avoid it. Who wants to get hit in the head? There were times when I couldn't avoid it, and in those situations the next best option was to try to meet the guy with the crown of my helmet (just the like players in the NFL study) and hit him harder than he hit me. I'm confident that most football players go through the same decision tree. Nowhere in that tree is there an option that says, "If all else fails, try to hit him with the side of your head." So it is safe to assume that players who get hit in the side of the head don't do it by choice, and from that we can conclude they don't see the hit coming—that's why they call it a "blindside" hit. In fact, that's exactly what the NFL found in its batch of thirty-one hits, writing, "The typical impact involved a player running to-ward another player, who was generally unaware of the closing angle."[43]

This is important for two reasons. First, if the athlete didn't see the hit coming, then he wasn't braced for it. Bracing for a hit—flexing the muscles of the body and especially the neck—allows those parts of the body to ab-sorb some force, reducing the amount that reaches the brain. Second, a hit to the side of the head is more likely to cause those rotational forces that aren't protected by a helmet.

Dr. Cantu, the vice president of NOCSAE, told me, "The theory behind the 'Revolution' is that if you build a helmet that's a little bit bigger, especially in the temple area, and padded more thickly, then you'll reduce force more than you would if you had thinner padding and not so big an outer shell. That theory is good for blows that go right to the temple, but that's it." If hits to the temple are usually blindside hits that cause rotational injuries, I question whether adding padding and thickness would make any measurable difference whatsoever. (It might be more effective to add those round mirrors that let you to see around corners.)

The other major design change to the Revolution was to increase the protection on the chin, adding more shell and padding in order to reduce the concussions caused by hits to that area. That's a logical change, but since the NFL study showed that only about 10 percent of the concussions it recorded were due to shots in this area, even if adding more plastic shell worked, it would make little overall difference.[44]

The major change in the Schutt DNA helmet was to replace the standard inflatable air sacs with a new type of "shock-absorbing material" called "Skydex."[45] The most curious remark about the Schutt DNA comes from Schutt's own research director, Larry Maddux. He claimed, "The pads absorb shock better than a much thicker layer of foam, leaving room for traditional padding to make the helmet more comfortable."[46] In the words of Dr. Cantu, helmets are "not even close" to reducing force enough to prevent concussions. If Skydex works so well, why wouldn't Schutt put so much in there that it's coming out of the ear holes, rather than focusing on "comfort padding"?

We can conclude from Maddux's statement that in modern helmet manufacturing, there is a clear trade-off between safety and comfort. When just two major manufacturers control more than 90 percent of the market, designs are based as much on capitalism as on science. If one helmet is noticeably less comfortable than the other, no one will want to wear it. Based on my research, I have a hard time telling whether comfort or safety is a higher priority for these manufacturers.

That argument became a focal point of a recent lawsuit against Riddell.[47] In 1995, Jose Rodriguez, a football player at Los Fresnos High School in California, suffered a subdural hematoma that left him in a permanent vegetative state. While trying to stay out of the legalities of the case,

I want to emphasize a few key points. The Rodriguez family sued because they believed that the helmet Jose was wearing was not the best design Riddell could have made at the time. They claimed that Riddell had in its possession better force-absorbing foam in 1995 than the one it had put in Jose's helmet, and had it been used instead, Jose would have been safer. A biomechanical expert testified on behalf of the Rodriguez family, saying that in 1995, Riddell could have produced a safer helmet using a higher ratio of energy-absorbing padding to comfort padding. Riddell's response was that the design wasn't practical. The Riddell helmet designer argued that players wouldn't wear a helmet if the company had removed its soft comfort cushioning and replaced it with harder, less comfortable energy-absorbing foam. Sound familiar?

Before 2006, there was no way to be sure if the newer helmet styles were better or worse than the older models. Then, in February of that year, a study was published in *Neurosurgery* that claimed that the Riddell Revolution decreased the risk of concussion over older models by 31 percent.[48] This made the headlines. It seemed like a cut and dry issue—Hooray! The Revolution reduces concussions! But the media didn't mention certain details of the study which cast an incredible amount of doubt on its integrity—including that Riddell had funded the study, and that its vice president of research and product development was one of its authors.

Luckily you don't have to take my word for it, because the peer reviewers tore the study to shreds. Dr. Cantu, who is on the editorial board of *Neurosurgery*, wrote a scathing review: "This article, in my opinion, suffers from a serious, if not fatal, methodological flaw." That fatal flaw is that the designers of the study chose to compare brand-new Riddell Revolution helmets to whatever older models the school district in the study was using. Dr. Cantu continued, "As Vice President of the National Operating Committee on Standards for Athletic Equipment (NOCSAE), the organization that makes the certification standards for football helmets and other athletic equipment, I am aware, as is the author of this article employed by Riddell, that new helmets test to a higher severity index level than older helmets. New helmets, out of the box before receiving the thousands of hits that they will incur on ensuing seasons, often test significantly below the 1200 severity index that they must pass. Then, with each year's passage of time, their abilities to attenuate acceleration forces decline. That is the reason for the requirement of helmet reconditioning and recertification after a period of years in use . . . It would be expected that if the newer Riddell helmets, therefore, are being compared against helmets that are significantly older, that the older helmet would not perform to as high a degree as the newer helmet. That is why today when parents or athletes ask me which is the best helmet to wear, I tell them I don't know which brand is best, but I know that a new helmet will be better than an old helmet and if recurring concussions are a concern that they should equip themselves with a new helmet."

The authors of the Riddell study weakly defended their choice to compare old and new helmets by writing, "Reports issued annually by NAERA (the National Athletic Equipment Reconditioners Association) to its membership indicate that properly reconditioned and recertified football helmets do not diminish in measured performance when compared to newly manufactured helmets." At best, that statement is partly true, and it's certainly not the whole truth. Another peer reviewer, USC Athletic Trainer Russ Romano, blasted that defense. "Certification of used helmets usually is recommended every two years," he wrote. "The reconditioning process involves a visual inspection, and only four percent of the batch actually undergoes laboratory testing. The decrease in concussion rates [found in the Revolution group] may be owing to newer materials instead of newer technology."

The most telling review was from Dr. Michael Levy, who wrote that it was "problematic" that a Riddell vice president would suggest that reconditioned helmets are as good as new helmets when, "Riddell suggests that its helmets be retired after ten years of use." Peer reviewer Dr. Art Day summed it up perfectly when he wrote, "Most importantly, each of the authors has a business relationship with either the computerized neurocognitive testing equipment company (Im-PACT) or the helmet manufacturer (Riddell) that were being evaluated. This fact represents a substantial conflict of interest, and the results should be interpreted accordingly." Amen.

▼▼▼

Occasionally, a company will develop an interesting and innovative new football helmet. In his role as NOCSAE vice president, Dr. Cantu has seen a range of designs—from one that used Velcro to attach Styrofoam to the top of a helmet to a system that deployed an airbag collar to prevent neck fractures. But perhaps the most interesting was a radical design by a company called Protec. Its helmet was intended to prevent broken necks, but it also happened to work incredibly well to reduce concussions. Due to safety and liability concerns, the Protec system never saw action in a game, and Protec's experience reveals how those two barriers may prevent innovative, new designs from getting out of the laboratory and onto the playing field.

"This system created an indestructible head, neck, and thorax football player," Dr. Cantu remembered. "It was made of fiberglass; the athlete actually wore two helmets. The inner helmet was worn directly on the head and it had no hard outer shell—it was just an energy attenuating substance, and not very thick. They didn't need to put any hard shell on it because what was going to protect the head from any of those issues was going to be the outer construct.

"The outer helmet looked like a regular football helmet, but was so huge that it almost looked more like a helmet that people would wear to walk on the moon. It was so grotesquely oversized that it was unreal. It had a facemask, and literally swiveled and locked like a deep-sea diver's helmet. It locked on shoulder pads, which consisted of a one-piece shoulder pad with a front and back flak jacket. Envision this little helmeted head inside this large outer shell helmet; the inner helmet does not touch the outer helmet. You can make the analogy that the inner helmet was like the inner liner in a regular football helmet, and the outer helmet was like the outer liner of an existing helmet—only now you've got an air pocket of several inches in between.

"Because there were a couple inches of air between the hard outer helmet and inner helmet, the forces that were being transmitted to the inner helmet were tremendously dampened. So as a byproduct of this, the neck and the head were both protected. The blows that were taken by the helmet essentially bypassed the neck and went directly to the shoulder pad, greatly attenuating by about 80 percent the forces that otherwise would have been taken by the neck and head. I never saw it tested on the severity index, but you probably would get below the magic number of 300 with this concept and therefore prevent concussion.

"The first question we asked was, 'Could a receiver see a ball wearing this stuff?' The outer construct didn't move except when the whole body turned sideways. So the company actually did some football drills and videotaped them, and, by God, he could do it. They taped a receiver catching passes and doing drills, which looked funny when you saw the size of that outer helmet, but it worked. The athlete could see back over his shoulder.

"The NCAA looked at this device, and I'll never forget it—it said, quite wisely, 'But what about the rest of the body?' This thing created an indestructible head, neck, and thorax football player. It was made of fiberglass. If you had people wearing these things they would become flying missiles from the waist up, essentially invulnerable to injury.

"That doesn't say what would happen below the flak jacket—to the abdomen, the pelvis, the knees, etc.—because these fiberglass objects would just crash into other parts of the body, probably shattering knee caps and rupturing spleens. So what the NCAA said was, 'This is very interesting, this protects the neck, and we're interested in that concept. But we're worried about the rest of the body, and we're also worried about it changing the way the sport would be played. If you think there's not much spearing and cut blocking going on now, you can imagine what there'd be with these things on. So for fear of injuries to other parts of the body that would be catastrophic, we will not approve this for use.'

"The NCAA went on to say, 'We won't sanction this unless studies are done that prove that it doesn't ruin the rest of the bodies of young men. And by the way, you have to pay for those studies. If you fund studies about the safety of this equipment to other parts of the body, then we'll look at it again when you present that data to us.' In essence, the NCAA was turning its back on these people who had invested their own money to do the engineering studies that showed the reduction of forces to the neck and reduction of forces to the head.

"The field testing of this stuff would have meant that Protec had to go to a league, and basically have the schools in the league agree that half of their players would wear this stuff, and half wouldn't. They would have had to outfit a number of high-school teams with the Protec gear, and then let them play against other teams that were willing to play against this gear while not wearing it.

"Only then would we see who didn't get a concussion, who didn't get a cervical spine injury and, by the way, who picked up lacerated spleens and shattered pelvises and knees and everything else. Also, the company would then have had to underwrite the liability if there were a lot of serious abdominal injuries or knee injures. If those injuries were shown to be directly due to wearing this equipment, then they could potentially be liable for having 'caused' those injuries. This put the company out of business because they couldn't fund those kinds of studies."

NOCSAE also avoided the responsibility of evaluating the Protec helmet. Dr. Cantu continued, "NOCSAE squirmed out of it by virtue of a technical loophole. It just so happened that I was there. NOCSAE certifies helmets by using a drop test, but it couldn't apply that test to this double-helmeted construct. You can drop the outer helmet from 60 inches, and you can drop the inner helmet from 60 inches, but you can't drop the inner inside the outer without it being in a body. It would be just rattling around in there. So NOCSAE couldn't test the hard outer fiberglass outfit.

"However, it did test the inner helmet, and believe it or not, that little inner helmet made of advanced materials passed NOCSAE standards! So the inner helmet could have gotten the NOCSAE seal. But the laws say that the NOCSAE seal must be visible on a football helmet. With that little helmet being inside the big one, you wouldn't see the seal on it when you wore the outer one. So 'technically' they were in violation of NOCSAE rules, and NOCSAE got around certifying them on that technicality. So essentially what was an interesting concept—I admit that that particular model of it doesn't really work—went by the boards for those reasons."

The major lesson to be learned from this story is that even if a new, innovative helmet could theoretically eliminate concussions from the game, it would be extremely hard to prove that it worked in an industry that has been burned by liability and litigation. In 1975, there were fourteen helmet manufacturers. That year a 19-year-old football player suffered an on-field injury that left him a quadriplegic. He sued the helmet manufacturer and was awarded a settlement of $5.3 million, which was later paid as a $3 million out-of-court settlement. Right or wrong, this began a trend. Payouts from lawsuits against helmet manufacturers reached $22 million in 1981–1982, when the gross income of the entire industry was $20 million.[49] Companies became either bankrupt or left the business, leaving only five manufacturers by 1990, and three today. Any radical changes in helmet design would logically come from these three companies, but they are worried, rightfully so, about liability issues.

It was a risk for Riddell to release a new helmet design, but it apparently felt that the NFL concussion data offered enough protection to try to get a leg up in the market. It was a market ripe for change, because litigation had basically frozen any innovation for thirty years. Bike Athletic Company developed a new helmet in 1999, but it never caught on and Bike filed for bankruptcy in 2002.[50] It's curious that Bike's new helmet didn't succeed, as it was endorsed by the NFL Players Association.[51] Unfortunately for Bike, it wasn't endorsed by the NFL and Dr. Elliott Pellman. Pellman told the press that he was "worried that the new helmet does not provide adequate protection to the sides of players' heads and might make players more susceptible to concussions." The president of the firm that helped run the NFL concussion studies, Dr. James Newman, also tried to cast doubt on the Bike model, saying, "Our research is suggesting that NOCSAE tests are not rigorous enough, so that you couldn't assume this helmet would perform well at higher levels of contact." That was an odd criticism, and not really a knock on Bike, because the same thing could have been said about any helmet in 1999, even Riddell's.

The NFLPA charged, "The league is deliberately withholding results of Newman's study and purposely undermining the credibility of the Bike helmet because of the league's contractual affiliation with Riddell." Ah, I see now. Riddell pays the NFL so that Riddell can be the "Official Helmet of the NFL." The circus continued when *Newsday* reported, "Some NFL officials counter that they believe the union may have a financial relationship with Bike." In my humble opinion, no matter who was paying whom, the real loser in this battle was every football player in America.

▼▼▼

The first goal in solving football's concussion crisis is to reduce the number of concussions that players sustain. Unfortunately, neither rule changes nor improved helmet technology appears capable of this in the foreseeable future. A custom mouthpiece is getting attention from the media, spurred by a dentist who has outfitted some NFL players with his patented product, including many of the New England Patriots. Dr. Gerald Maher claims that his mouthpiece reduces concussions by properly aligning the jaw. I don't know if this specific product works, but I do know that no controlled study has ever found that a mouthpiece significantly reduces concussions. Dr. Maher only has anecdotal evidence to support his claims.

Perhaps it's impossible to attenuate all of the forces created by 300-pound men running into each other as hard as they can. The energy has to go somewhere, and as the Protec system showed, if it doesn't go into the brain, it will go into the body. Perhaps as armor continues to evolve, we will eventually have to consciously choose which parts of boys' bodies are most expendable.

However, there are still incredible strides to be made in improving the outcomes for children playing football today. Right now, only a small percentage of concussions are diagnosed, meaning that only a small number are treated by trained medical personnel. If we can just get kids to tell an adult when they get "dinged," perhaps we can reduce the risk of further brain damage from secondary impacts. Educational outreach will be the major catalyst for change, but convincing players to speak up when they have a concussion is no easy task.

CHAPTER *10*

Tell Me What's Wrong

Today, knowing what I know, would I consider taking myself out of the game because I thought I'd gotten a concussion? During the heat of battle, no, because when you're playing, you want to play. You're not out there to just take up space.

Harry Carson, 53, NFL Hall of Famer

Depending on the severity of a concussion, you may feel fine pretty quickly, even if you had a significant injury. I think that a lot of times guys want to go back in just because they feel fine, not knowing that there may be more to it than what they actually feel.

Frank Volpe, 26, former college football player

I think that if it were spelled out for players so that they understood the ramifications and how permanent it can be, then I've got to believe that a person who values his life, his health, and his family would be honest and report it. But it has to be presented to the players correctly. You can't say, "If you get a concussion you've got to let us know because you're going to miss two weeks." Well, why is this so important? Why is this so serious? Players don't know why. If they're told, and if they understand, then I guarantee we'll have greater cooperation.

Merril Hoge, 41, nine-year NFL veteran

I worry that if I tell somebody [about my head], it might end up not being anything. So if I feel like something keeps happening, or if it still hurts, I tell somebody. But if it's something that goes away, I just think, "Okay, it went away, I'm not going to make a big deal out of it."

Steve, 16, high-school football player

The concussion problem in football is often framed as a new problem. Most older players I spoke with said some variation of, "Back in my day, when we were knocked silly, the doctor would dust us off and throw us back in. Nobody knew any better." That statement implies that we didn't know that concussions were dangerous until recently, and that players receive better treatment today. While it is true that athletes receive better emergency treatment, a coach's diary written one hundred years ago made me question whether athletes are really better off today.

My former roommate Brian Daigle, who was also my teammate at Harvard, is a collector of Harvard football memorabilia. One afternoon a book in his bookcase caught my eye: *Big-Time Football at Harvard, 1905: The Diary of Coach Bill Reid*. I wondered how concussions were treated when the game was in its infancy, so I began reading the diary with an eye out for any discussion of head injuries. I was richly rewarded, as deaths caused by head injuries were central to the movement to ban the game in 1905. Bill Reid, the coach of one of the most prominent college football programs in the nation, was right in the middle of it. The fate of football was so grim that on November 22, 1905, the week of the Harvard-Yale game, the two schools engaged in a debate titled: "Resolved that the intercollegiate football in America is a detriment rather than a benefit."

When Union College halfback Harold Moore died of a cerebral hemorrhage in a game against New York University on November 25, 1905, the chancellor of NYU requested that they hold a conference to abolish or reform football. Only through the staunch support of men like President Theodore Roosevelt, Harvard class of 1880, did the reformists win.[1] Roosevelt saw football as a metaphor for life, saying, "Hit the line hard: Don't foul and don't shirk, but hit the line hard." And Harvard President Charles Eliot would write, "effeminacy and luxury are even worse evils than brutality."

Coach Reid kept a detailed account of the players' injuries throughout the season. I was immensely curious to see how concussions had been treated in such a brutal era—if at all. As incidence studies have proven, few concussions reach the attention of coaches today, so I wasn't sure that Coach Reid had even been aware of them. It turned out that Coach Reid had only known of one. But the way he and the team approached that concussion took me by surprise.

In his diary, Coach Reid wrote that team captain Dan Hurley began to act strangely ten days before the end of the season. The team doctor, Dr. Edward Nichols, was the first to notice and asked the coaching staff if they'd noticed Dan acting "a little queer in his mind."[2] Coach Reid had not, but promised "to keep a close eye on him from now on."[3]

Four days later, Dr. Nichols again said that he was worried that Dan Hurley was "a little out of his head."[4] Coach Reid resisted Dr. Nichol's diagnosis, writing, "None of us will believe this, but are all going to watch him carefully from now on." He continued, "What makes me uncomfortable about the thing is that the fellows who were in the Dartmouth game complained that Hurley was blaming men for not being where they ought to be, when, as a matter of fact, they were doing just what they ought to do."

Two days later, Coach Reid finally had a chance to sit down with Hurley. It was no longer possible to ignore Hurley's outrageous behavior. At the team lunch, Coach Reid noticed that Hurley "frequently repeated sentences that he had said two or three times one after the other, . Urging him as best I could, I was unable to get him to eat anything but prunes for lunch. . . . Besides this he was late at lunch and I could not seem to impress on him the necessity of promptness." Hurley's behavior began to border on the comical. He was held out of practice, but because he had yet to see a specialist, no one had thought to keep an eye on him outside of practice. That night, Coach Reid stopped by the athletic office and discovered that he'd just missed seeing Hurley there. Hurley had stopped by to order some tickets and "along with them had asked for a bowl of crackers and milk."[5] Coach Reid reported this to Dr. Nichols, who from then on made sure that someone always traveled with Hurley in order to "prevent possibility of accident through the chances of temporary insanity."[6]

When the specialist finally examined him, he ordered that Hurley be sent to bed immediately, and that he be kept under a doctor's watch. He also decided that Hurley wouldn't play in the Yale game. While Hurley's behavior was not the strangest I've come across, the reaction of his teammates was. In my experience, a player with a concussion is often ostracized by his teammates. With an "invisible injury," he's forgotten and replaced with someone who "can get the job done." But Hurley's teammates were so concerned for his well-being that they sent telegrams to his hospital room from the road by special wire no fewer than three times. That was a nice gesture, but the team took it to a whole new level when, on the way to the train, they sang the following song to Dan:

Here's to you Dan Hurley,
Here's to you my jovial soul,
Here's to you with all my heart,

And now we're in your company,
We'll have a drink before we part,
Here's to you Dan Hurley.

The Harvard team took the injury seriously on all fronts. Coach Reid was so concerned about the bad publicity from Hurley's "concussion on the brain" that he lied to a rally of two thousand boosters on the eve of "The Game," noting, "I then explained as best I could the reason for Hurley's inability to play, placing more emphasis on his leg than I did on his head. Since football is being severely criticized just at present, a case of concussion on the brain would be very serious."

Today, over a century later, the players, the media, and the fans seem desensitized to the seriousness of the same injury, despite our knowledge that concussions are a far more significant and permanent injury than was ever imagined in 1905. Dr. Nichols instituted a concussion rule during the 1905 season, and Coach Reid allowed the doctor to explain it to the athletes directly. The rule was:

> In case any man in any game got hurt by a hit on the head so that he did not realize what he was doing, his team mate should at once insist that time be called and that a doctor come onto the field to see what is the trouble, also that every man on the squad must make up his mind in case he gets hurt, to have a friend with him from the time an injury occurred until noon of the next day, to prevent any serious results from beginning without anybody being around.[7]

A study published in 2003 found that half the athletes at the University of Akron—students between the ages of 17 and 24—didn't know that a head injury is anything to worry about. How often do you think today's student-athletes hear a speech like Dr. Nichols'?

I captured a more typical modern experience when I interviewed a 16-year-old football player who had just finished his sophomore season. Steve had never been diagnosed with a concussion, but he admits that that probably has less to do with never having had one, and more to do with that fact that he's never talked to a trainer or doctor about a concussion when it happened. "Five or six times a season I get hit, and my vision gets blurry or I kind of black out," Steve said. Sometimes, after a game or practice, "it's just a headache and I'm kind of 'out of it.' Other times I have to go lie in bed, I can't concentrate on anything, and I just feel awful."

Steve has never mentioned his experiences to anyone because, "I figured it was going to go away, and it did go away—so I didn't think much of it. I wasn't aware of any risks. Nobody has ever talked to me about anything that could happen if I played through a concussion." While Steve's experience is unfortunate, it's benign compared to what happened to one of his team-mates. "Last year, one of my running backs wasn't doing too well after a hit," Steve began. "He didn't know where he was or what he was doing—he had to be told each play. He was still playing well because he was just that good, but he had to be told coming out of the huddle what to do. When he had the ball in his hands, he just ran like it was his nature and he still got to the end zone somehow.

"On the sideline, I saw the trainer give him some smelling salts. The trainer waved them back and forth under his nose, but he didn't flinch. He couldn't smell anything, he was so out of it. The trainer was so shocked that I saw him smell them himself to make sure they were working. The trainer pulled his head away real fast because they smelled horrible. Then the trainer put them back near the kid's nose, but, again, the kid couldn't smell any-thing. The trainer threw them on the ground after about five minutes. I picked them up to smell them. The smell was horrible—I was amazed that the kid couldn't smell that.

I asked, "So, what happened next?" I was assuming that the player's hel-met was taken away, and that possibly an ambulance was called.

"The kid kept playing. The trainer didn't really want him to, but the kid said, 'I'm going back in, so there's nothing you can do about it.'"

Where is Dr. Nichols when you need him? Only time will tell if the ill-advised behavior of Steve and his teammate will lead to neurological prob-lems in the future.

▼▼▼

If we want to help players avoid the negative consequences of concussions, our top priority must be to diagnose a higher percentage of concussions. This means educating players, first teaching them how to know when a con-cussion has actually occurred. Definitively diagnosing a concussion is not like diagnosing other injuries. A concussion can't be seen on an X-ray, and MRI and computed tomography (CT) scans aren't useful in diagnosing the vast majority of concussions. Dr. Chae explained to me, "Only in the most severe cases of concussion can you see some evidence of injury on an MRI. The only thing that you want to do after concussion is make sure that the person does not develop a subdural hematoma. That can be done with a CT scan on the head right away."

So, sideline medical personnel diagnose a concussion by subjectively looking for symptoms that represent the loss of brain function. This is an inexact science at best. As former college football player Frank Volpe said, "If you black out and you're puking all night, it's easy to say to yourself, 'Okay, I've probably had a concussion,' but how do you really know what's wrong when most of the time the people who are diagnosing you don't really know? They can shine a light in your eyes and say, 'Your pupils look fine,' but what if you have blurry vision? What does that mean?

"It's like it's somebody's opinion whether or not you had one. It's not possible to do tests on a concussion, like you can do on a knee to find out if there's a torn ligament. A lot of times guys feel fine, and there's no way to really know whether they've had a concussion or not." Trainers rely on symptom lists, but when those lists are broken down, it becomes clear that a concussion diagnosis depends considerably on what the athlete tells the trainer.

When concussion symptoms are divided into two groups—those that the trainer or any outside observer can identify, and those that depend on the player's speaking up—the list is heavily weighted toward the latter. The following list uses the NFL's definition of concussion from the journal *Neurosurgery*:

> A traumatically induced alteration in brain function manifested by an alteration of awareness or consciousness, including but not limited to a

Observable	Not Often Observable
loss of consciousness, seizure	"ding" sensation of being dazed or stunned sensation of "wooziness" or "fogginess" amnesic period

. . . and by symptoms commonly associated with post-concussion syndrome, including

Observable	Not Often Observable
loss of balance	persistent headaches
syncope (LOC)	vertigo (dizziness)
near-syncope	light-headedness
	unsteadiness
	cognitive dysfunction
	memory disturbances
	hearing loss
	tinnitus (ringing in the ears)
	blurred vision
	diplopia (double vision)
	visual loss
	personality change
	drowsiness
	lethargy
	fatigue
	inability to perform usual daily activities

Even observable symptoms aren't always caught. One study found that 24 percent of players experiencing a loss of consciousness didn't tell anyone.[8]

Concussion diagnosis is flawed because of this dependence on the player to report his symptoms. As Dr. Delaney explained, "We have all these new technologies to treat concussions, but the problem is that we're still dependent on the player telling us, 'I just don't feel right.'" To make things worse, players rarely have easy access to the medical experts to whom they would need to say, "I just don't feel right." I was shocked to find that only about 30 to 33 percent of all high schools have a certified athletic trainer on staff. In poor districts like those in Chicago's public school system, just 2 percent of high schools have trainers at practice, and only 9 percent have them at games.[9] [10] Even when a school has a trainer, they have to cover multiple sports, so they aren't always near the football team during practice. This makes it even more difficult for players to talk to them about any symptoms.

Because of certain characteristics that are unique to the sport of football, this "player dependence" makes trainers virtually helpless to diagnose concussions without the help of the athlete.

A discussion with a former basketball player opened my eyes to this rarely discussed problem.[11] Basketball concussions are rarely missed by anyone watching the game, because everyone in the arena can see the players' faces. The look on a concussed athlete's face is often the first indication that something is wrong. In football, the player's face is hidden behind a helmet and facemask. In basketball, the court is small, so the athlete is never too far from the trainer or coach, and they can see subtle changes in his behavior. In football, the trainer is usually at least 30 yards away. In basketball, the game is continuous, so a drop-off in play is easily noticed. In football, a play lasts five seconds, and then there are thirty seconds until the next play. According to one player survey, 22 percent of concussions have symptoms that last less than five minutes.[12] Since no one outside the huddle may notice, it's fairly easy for an athlete to keep playing with a mild concussion. The player may even recover enough on the field to hide the injury by the time he reaches the sideline.

There's more: In basketball, collisions are memorable because they're so rare. In a football game, there are too many collisions per play to monitor them. In a practice, collisions occur in small groups all over the field. Even the most vigilant trainer or coach is guaranteed to miss things. Often the only person watching one specific football player on every play is that player's parent in the stands.

But even those parents are at a disadvantage, because they are incapable of spotting one of the most common external sign of concussion in football, the "blown assignment." Only the coach knows if a player has zigged when he should have zagged. Even the trainer doesn't have that knowledge. The coach is the only person who can recognize that telltale sign, but he's neither trained nor expected to diagnose concussions.

Diagnosing concussions is made more difficult because in many cases there is only a short window of time during which the symptoms exist. Player surveys reveal that in 50 percent of concussions, the symptoms last less than two hours, and in 72 percent they last less than one day. This means that concussions must be diagnosed when they happen. If no adult sees the concussion occur, and the player is able to finish the game, that player will have little incentive to mention the experience after the game because his symptoms will have disappeared. Dr. Cantu sums it up: "Unless kids take themselves out of the contests, there's no way to know that they've been mildly impaired. It's only when they're so impaired that they're missing plays, missing assignments, walking into the wrong huddle, etc. that outside observers know something is wrong. Obviously, that happens much less often, and nobody is going to miss that."

▼▼▼

So, we have to rely on kids to voluntarily report any concussion symptoms. This system isn't working today, because only between 1 and 10 percent of concussions are diagnosed, and 94 percent of football players with headaches continue to play.[13] To increase the reporting rate, we need to understand *why* players aren't speaking up.

Twenty-year professional and former Heisman Trophy winner Doug Flutie has had his share of concussions, and his experience highlights the *two subsets* of players who don't say anything—those who don't speak up *on purpose*, and those who are knocked too silly to know that anything is wrong. "It's drilled into kids' heads from day one that if they can walk, they can play," Doug told me. "We have to undo that with concussions." I met Doug at a charity basketball tournament in Boston that benefits the Doug Flutie Jr. Foundation for Autism. (Thanks to the generosity of the Shad Nation—who funded my basketball team—we won the 2006 championship, and I felt that earned me the right to ask Doug about his experience.)

"I had two major concussions," Doug said. "The first was in college in a game against Rutgers. I was kneed in the head, and immediately dazed. But I didn't really know anything was wrong. I went back into the game and went four for four with a touchdown pass, but when I went out for the huddle the next time, I couldn't remember how to run the play we were calling. My teammates had to call timeout and walk me off the field. When I watched the film, I saw that even while I was going four for four, I was throwing the ball to guys I would never usually throw it to. They weren't my normal reads.

"My worst concussion was in San Diego. When I got hit, my head was driven into the turf. I kind of blacked out, but I don't think I lost consciousness. When the trainers got to me, I remember sitting on the field telling them that I felt fine, but warning them that in a minute or two I'd be out of it. That's what I learned from the earlier concussions. As soon as you get it, you're fine, but slowly your brain starts to swell, or whatever, and then things get worse before they get better."

Flutie's personal experience taught him that even if the injury is mild, it's sometimes difficult for a concussed player to realize that something is wrong. "The problem with these concussions is that when you get it, you feel fine," he told me. "You can live in the moment. But thirty seconds later, you can't remember what happened, and then you're back to living in the moment again. You can't tell *as an individual* that something is wrong." Flutie also knows that even if a player is aware of his concussion, he still may not speak up. "The problem is that kids have the same competitive drive as the professionals do. So they're not going to want to go out when, in the moment, they feel fine."

The players who are knocked silly are usually the players who get diagnosed because they either can't function or, like in Doug's case, they act so strangely that their teammates say something. But most of the players who *can* play *choose* to continue to play. Thanks to a few innovative studies, we now know why.

McCrea and colleagues found that the principle reason players don't speak up is that they don't think that the injury is serious enough. This finding has been confirmed by at least one other study.[14] [15]

Reasons Why Concussions Are Not Reported*

Did not think it was serious enough	66.4%
Did not want to leave game	41.0%
Did not know it was a concussion	36.1%
Did not want to let down teammates	22.1%

* Players could give more than one reason.

Why don't kids think that this injury is serious enough to merit the attention of a trainer? I think one clue that's overlooked is that players know a trainer cannot make the concussion feel any better. If I sprain my ankle, I tell the trainer. He tapes it up so that I can play better, ices it so that it feels better, and rehabs it so that I can return to full-strength more quickly. But an athlete knows that if he tells the trainer that he has a concussion, the trainer can't make it hurt less or heal faster. A player who is unaware of the risks of continuing to play with a concussion believes that he has nothing to gain by speaking up. On the flip-side, he has a lot to lose because the trainer may pull him out—an especially frustrating outcome if the athlete feels that he can still compete.

With that in mind, we have to make players aware of the risks of playing through a concussion. This educational effort will be an uphill battle. Knowledge of the injury is so poor that one recent study found that 92 percent of athletes and coaches believed that a "bellringer" or a "dinger" was a different injury from a concussion.[16] But education alone won't change everyone's behavior. Merril Hoge believes, "If you explain the truth to these players, you're going to get the people who'll immediately respond, and then you'll have people say, 'I'm not going do that.'"

The players who don't get onboard are probably those in McCrea's survey who said that they hid concussions because they "did not want to leave the game" and "did not want to let down their teammates." In my interviews with dozens of football players of all age groups, almost everyone mentioned those two reasons. To overcome this behavior, we have to understand their deeper motivations.

The justifications that the players gave for "not wanting to leave the game" essentially fell into three distinct buckets: football's injury culture, fear of competition, and fear of backlash from coaches.

Football's Injury Culture

Football has a culture of toughness. Most players learned the same approach toward injury—the mantra mentioned by Doug Flutie: "If you can walk, you can play." Others told me they were taught that "pain is weakness leaving the body," that "you play until someone has to carry you off the field," or simply that "you never take yourself out of the game." One high-school football player told me, "It's been pounded into my head, and probably pounded into the heads of several thousand football players across the country, that pain is weakness, pain is something you can deal with. You can always push harder, so basically, if it's absolutely impossible to run, then you're hurt. I guess that's usually where I draw the line. But if it's pain and you can still function, you play."

I eventually learned to play through pain. In my junior year of high school I fractured a bone in my hand in the second quarter of a game. I continued to play. By the third quarter, the pain and swelling were so great that I was only using my right hand, while trying to protect my left from any contact whatsoever. During a timeout, I was near the sideline getting defensive signals from a coach, and I said to him, "I don't need to come out, but just so you know, I've hurt my hand and I'm playing one-handed out there." He looked at me, blinked once, nodded, and proceeded to give me the defensive call. I think the coach quickly figured that I was more effective with one hand than my backup was with two.

I cannot completely knock learning to play through pain. A successful player has to play through pain and injury at some point in his career, and a successful team needs a lot of players who are willing to do that. It builds character. As one former player told me, "Football was the time of your life when you went beyond what you thought your physical capabilities were." But until we teach players that this attitude should only apply to injuries below the neck, we're exposing them to needless risk.

Competition

Other players feared losing playing time or their starting position if they played an active role in removing themselves from play. More than one athlete specifically mentioned Lou Gehrig's famous 2,130 consecutive-games streak. Most sports fans know that, according to legend, the streak began when Willy Pipp—the New York Yankees first baseman Gehrig replaced—asked for a day off because of a headache. Pipp never took the field again for the Yankees.

Some players rush back to play because they're worried about appearing injury prone. My former teammate Anthony Ackil said, "I'm pretty sure I had a concussion my freshman year of college. I tore my hamstring the first day of my freshman year, and it took me a week and a half to get back. My first day back, I remember this play where I smacked my head against somebody. For the next two weeks, every time I would step down my head would hurt. I played horribly during that time. I didn't tell anybody because I didn't want to sit out again after having sat out with my hamstring injury. I just thought that if I was hurt again, it would look like I would always be hurt."

Former college fullback Frank Volpe played with this fear. He said, "The only reason I got the opportunity to play as a freshman was because one of the upperclassmen got hurt. In the second half against Bucknell, I got a pretty good lick. I'm out there playing with blurry vision, and I'm thinking, 'I can barely see 10 feet in front of me. What am I going to do?' Then I thought, 'I've been waiting for this opportunity for a long time. I'm not going to have this opportunity again, because if that senior goes back in there and does just well enough to not get taken out of a game, I'm not playing anymore.'

"It was the fear of what would happen if I wasn't on the field, because I was always one of those people who thought that, if given the opportunity, I could do as well as anyone else. I wasn't as big as everybody else, but I knew that I would put myself in positions where the odds of success were pretty good. I knew that when we played Bucknell that day in the rain, that if I came out of there, and someone else went in, I may never get another opportunity like that again."

Frank believes that his shortsighted behavior led to permanent damage. He explained, "To this day, about twenty minutes to a half-hour after some of my workouts, my vision slowly starts to go. It's almost like I'm looking through a broken glass. I can't see or focus on anything. It usually lasts about a half-hour to forty-five minutes, and is followed up by an intense headache that usually lasts overnight into the next day."

Coaching

Other players didn't want to voluntarily leave the game because of explicit or implicit pressure from their coaches. High-school player Nick Fisher remembers, "If you take yourself out, that would indicate to the coach that you didn't really want to be there. Coaches see it as a sign of weakness, and that you don't want to play. You've got to play while you're hurt to prove to them that you really want to play."

Most football players aren't born to ignore pain and injuries—they learn it. The football field is the classroom, and the coaches are the teachers. The question coaches usually rely on, one that I imagine every player can quote verbatim, is, "Are you injured, or are you hurt?" Injured implies that you can't continue; hurt means you can carry on. Now, I don't think coaches are necessarily bad guys because they're trying to toughen players up. Football isn't tiddlywinks, and a lot of us owe the best parts of our characters to what we learned from the game and from coaches. But sometimes the pressure to play through an injury can be enormous. During my freshman spring at Harvard, the football team was invited to Japan to play the national champion Kyoto University football team in a goodwill game. We went a week early to tour the country, visiting the Imperial Palace, meditating with Buddhist monks on a mountaintop, and going out for Karaoke with the Kyoto football players. We also practiced every day. Early in the week I strained my hip flexor on the turf at Kawasaki Stadium. The hip flexor is the muscle that lifts the thigh forward and up, so it was difficult and painful to run.

The trainers recommended that I take a few days off. (One of the dangers of playing through that kind of muscle pull, besides damaging it further, is that it causes you to limp, which can lead to further and more serious injuries.) I was comfortable with that advice because I knew I'd be useless on the field if I couldn't run. My defensive line coach did not agree.

He approached me in the hotel lobby the next morning and asked, "Can you practice today?" I said, "The trainer says I should take a few days off." He looked me in the eye and said, "I didn't ask what the trainer said. I asked *you* if you can practice today." Now, I was only 18 at the time, and didn't immediately see where this was going. I said, "I don't understand the question." He got frustrated and blurted, "If someone came up to you right now and held a gun to your head, would you be able to run away?" As he asked, he made a gun with his thumb and index finder and pointed it at me in case I didn't understand what he meant. I practiced that day. I have no doubt that this coach toughened me up, and my change of attitude toward injury contributed to my successful career. Unfortunately, I don't remember being told that this new philosophy should never be applied to injuries above the shoulders. A coach who is not educated about the risks of concussions can be dangerous to his players.

One of the studies that looked at why players didn't report concussions found that the *coach's knowledge and attitude toward head injuries* significantly influenced whether or not players reported them to medical personnel.[17] A 14-year-old player told me, "My starting quarterback got about five concussions last season. Coach calls him 'Baby' now because his head's so soft. He's a tough kid, though. He kept playing when he could, or when the doctor would let him. But he'd just get better, come back, and get another."

Some of this pressure is institutionalized. In many programs, injured athletes are forced to watch practice in full pads and helmets while wearing a yellow or pink jersey over their regular practice jersey. We're told that this makes things more "efficient" and "safe," allowing a coach to know who's injured, and preventing other players from accidentally running into the injured guys. In reality, the jersey functions much like the "Scarlet Letter." The player might as well wear a flashing neon sign that says, "I'm soft."

To be fair, let's not forget that coaches are under pressure to win games. They walk a fine line between taking care of their players' long-term health and keeping their jobs. Even high-school coaches are rewarded for winning and fired for losing. If we give them a personal stake in putting the best team on the field, we shouldn't be surprised that some will do whatever they can to keep guys on the field, especially when they only appear to have a headache.

Letting Teammates Down

The other justification players gave for hiding concussions was that they "did not want to let their teammates down." This is a different problem, and not easily overcome by education. Imagine that you're a 15-year-old football player. A player falls on your teammate's ankle, and he's rolling on the ground in pain. He limps off the field with the help of teammates. The trainers tape up his foot to make it immobile. He limps back onto the field to a roar of respect from the crowd. You see him gritting his teeth to play through the pain. On the next play, you get hit in the head. Your vision goes a little blurry, and you have a mild headache. No one can tell that anything is wrong with you. Do you shake hands with your injured teammate and say, "Good luck, I'm done for the day," or do you keep fighting alongside him, knowing that he's in more pain than you are? Even with what I know about concussions, a part of me can't help but think how admirable it is to keep fighting alongside that teammate.

I was discussing this issue with Brian Howard, one of my best friends and the guy I lined up next to for four years at Harvard. He summed it up perfectly: "Sure, there's pressure to not report concussions. You want a teammate who will line up every play, even when he's messed up. You know you can count on that guy. If you think that guy isn't going to play hard, or will pull himself out when he's hurt, down, or not 100 percent, then you don't want that guy lining up next to you." To solve this problem, I think it will be up to players to convince each other that it's okay to rest with a concussion, because it's simply a different injury with far more serious consequences.

As we fight this uphill battle to radically change the behavior of these young men, let's not forget the pressure of the moment. It's not uncommon for a competitive player—like Wayne Chrebet—to do everything in his power to stay in a game after suffering a concussion, and then publicly say the next day that he regretted his decision. We usually chalk that bad decision up to "the heat of the moment," but it turns out that those poor decisions actually have biological roots.

Behavioral economics is an academic field of study that's quickly gaining credibility. It helps explain why people consistently make what appear to be irrational decisions.[18] In the subfield of neuroeconomics, researchers are using MRIs to investigate cerebral blood flow patterns during decision making. They've found that the brain has two key subsystems involved in decision making. The limbic and paralimbic system controls emotional responses on an unconscious level, and the analytic system, which is centered in the parietal and frontal cortexes, controls calculated future-oriented decisions.

Studies have found that when an individual makes a decision that affects the present moment (like when he suffers a concussion in a game), if there is an emotional component (like not wanting to let down his teammates) and the limbic system shows activity, the emotional response will dominate the analytic response (which would be to rest the concussion), and the person will be more likely to make a decision that goes against his conscious long-term goals.

▼▼▼

When you combine a never-quit attitude with multiple concussions, you can get a perfect storm of dangerous behavior. I played with a guy at Harvard whose lack of regard for his body forced him to retire prematurely, and his experience reveals just how much we have to overcome to make the game safer. (Months after our interview he asked that I not use his name, so "Mike" is a pseudonym. He plans to have a career in politics and doesn't want to be pigeon-holed as someone who has brain damage. Other athletes turned down interviews immediately for similar concerns.)

"My first concussion was during my senior year of high school," Mike told me. "I made a tackle and my eyesight went completely to hell. I couldn't see anything; everything I saw was slanted up to the right. I remember standing on the field, looking over to the sidelines trying to get the signals in, but I couldn't see what the coach was doing. I kept yelling at the coach, 'I can't see you! I can't see you! I can't see you!' He screamed back at me, 'What are you talking about?' I finally told another linebacker to take the signal and call out the play. He called out the play, and then I had him line me up. He lined me up, they ran the next play, the running back got the ball . . . and ran right by me. I didn't even see him run by. Eventually he got tackled, they ran out the clock and the half was over.

"I came off to the sideline and the coach started yelling at me, saying, 'What the hell were you doing?' and I said, 'I just couldn't see him.' Again he said, 'What are you talking about?' and I said, 'I can't see right now.' The trainer, who was actually one of the best trainers I've ever had, came over along with some doctors. They put me through all the tests on the sideline—count back from 100 by 7's and all that. I did fine. They asked what the last quarter was, and I said, 'Second.' They said, 'What's the score?' I said, 'We're losing.' I got all that stuff right and they said, 'What's wrong?' and I said, 'My head's killing me and I can't see.' So they said, 'Take five minutes and see if you can regain your sight.' So I tried to lie down on the bench, but I got up, went to the bathroom and threw up for about five minutes. When I came back to the bench to lie down, I could see again.

"So the doctors let me go back out there, and I played the rest of the game. After the game my head hurt like hell. When I woke up the next day it still hurt, but since we had won, I didn't think much about it and I went on playing." Mike's concussion problems continued through college. Sometimes he just adjusted his chinstrap and kept playing, and other times he would get vision problems and would have to come out to be evaluated by the trainers. But the more experience with concussions he had, the more he resisted the tests.

Mike said, "I think that most people who have suffered a concussion memorize the test. I knew the test. They asked me what the score was, what the quarter was, how much time was left, etc. During one test I was facing the scoreboard, so I had all the answers right in front of me, like an open-book quiz. I can still count backwards by sevens today." But since he couldn't always fake the answers to the test, and he didn't want to waste time taking it, he did what he had to do to stay on the field.

His final concussion occurred in the fourth quarter of an important game. "Same old thing—I got hit in the head again and got a concussion," he recalled. "Some of the guys knew about my previous head problems, and I remember looking over at them in the huddle. They were looking back at me, knowing that I'd gotten hit. I said to them, 'Don't you say a damned thing. Don't tell anyone. I can make it.'"

That concussion proved to be the last straw. "For the next seven months I had continuous vision problems," he said. "I kept seeing sparkles in the upper left area of my vision. No one really knew what it was. I was suffering really bad headaches, I still do today. Meanwhile, school was going on, so I was having problems. I went into the college's disability office. They helped me petition to take only two classes, and they okay'd it because I couldn't handle the workload. I was fortunate enough to have had professors that understood, telling me things like, 'Take as much time as you need. What you're going through sounds awful, so let me know if I can be of help.'"

As the next season approached, Mike had to decide whether to play again. "My doctors said, 'You really might want to consider not playing.' After some thought I told the coach that I wasn't coming back. It was really hard. It was even harder to tell my teammates that I wasn't coming back, but a lot of them said, 'Good, take care of your body.' Your teammates often know more than the coaches and the trainers because they're your friends and they care about you. You tell them more than you're going to tell anyone else. So that was the end of my athletic career."

Mike feels that his experiences contributed to the memory problems that he has today. He revealed, "As I'm getting older, I'm starting to lose a lot of little memories. I don't know if it's because of age or because of my experience with the head injuries . . . that's a big question. Only time well tell. Right now I cannot survive without my calendar. If I don't write something down, it's likely that I'll forget it. I never, ever used to write anything down. I never wrote down one homework assignment, I never wrote down a date. Now, it's iffy."

▼▼▼

As Mike's experience teaches us, even if the trainer or coach does catch wind of the concussion, it's no guarantee that it will be properly diagnosed. Trainers and doctors diagnose concussions on the sideline through a clinical examination, testing the physical and mental abilities of the player. One common part of the examination is called the Standardized Assessment of Concussion (SAC).[19]

This test evaluates orientation, immediate memory, concentration, and delayed recall. It's scored by a point system, with the highest possible score being 30 points. In the "orientation" portion, the player must give the month, date, day of the week, year, and time within an hour. He gets one point for each correct answer. For "immediate memory," the doctor gives the player five words to remember, like key, orange, monkey, etc. The player must repeat them back three times, for a total of 15 points. For "concentration," the player has to repeat a string of digits, like 3-9-4, backwards. Each of the next three trials increases one digit in length, for a total of four points. Then, for one point, the player has to give the twelve months in reverse order. Finally, for the "delayed recall," the doctor asks the player to repeat those same five words from the beginning of the test one more time.

It's important for parents to realize that these sideline clinical tests may not be sensitive enough to catch any but the most severe injuries. A large study was performed using the SAC test, and some players were tested before the season to determine their uninjured "baseline" score.[20] The study revealed that unless the athlete was experiencing amnesia or loss of consciousness, the player's score at the time of concussion was very close to his preseason baseline, and after fifteen minutes his scores were virtually identical. Because the vast majority of concussions don't involve a loss of consciousness or amnesia, the test does not appear very practical—despite its widespread use.

Standardized Assessment of Concussion Score (out of 30 points)

Symptoms	Baseline	At Concussion	15 Minutes Later
No LOC/No Amnesia	27	24	26
Post-traumatic Amnesia	25	21	22
Loss of Consciousness	26	12	14

Based on the symptoms gained through whatever clinical testing is performed, the trainer will often give the concussion a grade in order to gauge its severity. The Cantu Evidence-Based Grading Scale is one of the more widely used systems, although there are over a dozen.[21]

Grade 1 (Mild)	No LOC, Post-traumatic amnesia <30 minutes, Post concussion signs/symptoms <24 hours
Grade 2 (Moderate)	LOC <1 minute or Post-traumatic amnesia ≥30 minutes or Post concussion signs/symptoms ≥ 24 hours <7 days
Grade 3 (Severe)	LOC ≥ 1 minute or Post-traumatic amnesia ≥24 hours or Post concussion signs/symptoms ≥7 days

The idea of grading concussions at the time of injury is losing steam. Some doctors, including Dr. Cantu, are beginning to advocate not grading the concussion until the symptoms have disappeared.[22] This is a logical step, considering the unpredictable nature of these injuries, and is covered in greater depth in the next chapter.

What Parents Can Do

To properly address a health concern of this magnitude, there must be practical reforms on multiple levels to increase reporting rates. The first step is to educate players and their parents. While some may think that this responsibility lies with schools, the statistics show that it may be primarily a parental responsibility. More than two out of three schools don't employ a certified athletic trainer, and studies show that after a trainer, players are just as likely to tell their parents about an injury as they are their coach.[23] Parents may need to sit down with their child and explain what a concussion is, how it happens, and what it means to the child's health. Familiarizing oneself with the symptom list used by the National Athletic Trainer's Association is a good start. The symptoms include:

Blurred vision
Dizziness
Drowsiness
Excess sleep
Easily distracted
Fatigue
Feel "in a fog"
Feel "slowed down"
Headache
Inappropriate emotions
Irritability
Loss of consciousness
Loss of orientation
Memory problems
Nausea
Nervousness
Personality change

Poor balance/coordination
Poor concentration
Ringing in ears
Sadness
Seeing stars
Sensitivity to light
Sensitivity to noise
Sleep disturbance
Vacant stare/glassy eyed
Vomiting

Parents should then be prepared to discuss with their child what an athlete can expect to feel after the injury. (The experiences in this book provide a great jumping-off point.) Parents must acknowledge that an athlete may not want to tell anybody about the concussion for fear of embarrassment, or for the many other reasons discussed earlier. Parents need to explain the risks of such behavior. They should also specifically discuss the athlete's concerns about losing his spot, repercussions from his coach, or not wanting to let his teammates down.

The second step is for parents to reach out to the trainers and coaches. They shouldn't assume that the trainer is up to date on the latest concussion management guidelines. The odds are he is not, as a recent study found that only 3 percent of trainers fully comply with the National Association of Athletic Trainers recommendations for concussions assessment and management.[24] Coaches need to be made aware of this information as well, because even if a coach has the best intentions, his attitude and awareness play an integral role in concussion diagnosis and treatment. (What he doesn't know about concussions can hurt your kid.)

Parents can expect some resistance from hardheaded coaches. In 1989, four Louisiana high-school football players sustained cervical spinal cord injuries—56 times the national rate.[25] Based on the assumption that players were being taught improper techniques, a training video on proper tackling was produced through support from the Louisiana Sports Medicine and Safety Advisory Council, the Louisiana Office of Public Health, Disability Prevention Program, the Children's Hospital of New Orleans, Tulane University, and the U.S. Centers for Disease Control and Prevention.[26] Copies of the video were distributed to every junior and senior high school and municipal athletic department in the state. The tape identified college and professional players who had suffered disabling neck injuries due to improper tackling, showed how their injuries had occurred, and demonstrated proper technique.[27]

When a follow-up study was performed to evaluate the players' knowledge of neck injuries, only 12 percent of the players had actually seen this free video.[28] When the coaches from the fourteen schools that refused to show the tape were reached for an explanation, three refused to be interviewed. The eleven others admitted to being aware of the tape. When asked why they hadn't shown it, five coaches responded that they hadn't found the time to show this short video. The other six expressed their concern that the video might make their players play less aggressively.

Whitey Baun, a former college player and current youth football coach, explains, "I've been coaching peewee football for eight years, and I've never had any training on concussions. The coaches are the ones who really need to know about this research. It's tough, because they don't know how serious it can be, but they're responsible for young kids. They have this attitude, 'Let's get him back in.' I've seen a guy get knocked silly. A doctor says, 'He really shouldn't go back in,' but the coach says, 'Oh no, he seems fine. He's good.' The coaches aren't trying to be mean, they just don't know any better."

Third, we would make great gains by applying the wisdom of Harvard's Dr. Nichols from a century ago. Dr. Nichols told the team, "In case any man in any game got hurt by a hit on the head so that he did not realize what he was doing, his team mate should at once insist that time be called and that a doctor come onto the field to see what is the trouble."[29] If we can convince athletes to make a pact with each other to alert a trainer, coach, or parent if a player is acting strangely in the huddle, on the sidelines, or after the game, we can remove the pressure of the "heat of the moment." Then it will be more difficult for concussions to slip through the cracks.

Frank Rochon, now age 34, played offensive line at St. Ignatius high school, a football powerhouse in Cleveland, Ohio. The captain of his team, Frank missed most of his senior year with a concussion. He sustained it in the preseason, but continued to play for about a month even though he couldn't remember playing in any of the games once they were over. He returned for a playoff game, where his center, Shawn, received a concussion in the third quarter. Instead of alerting the coaches and the trainer, Frank and his fellow offensive linemen told Shawn what to do and who to block for the rest of the game. "Take the tackle, Shawn! Get the linebacker, Shawn! The snap is on one!" they would yell.

Frank still feels a sense of guilt about the whole situation. He says, "In the huddle, we were constantly saying, 'Shawn, turn around; Shawn, pay attention; Come on, Shawn.' We forced him to stay in the game. We knew the guy was rung-up, we knew his head was gone—but we needed him out there for the rest of that game for a chance to win. We were just hoping that the programming was there so that Shawn would remember how to snap the ball, where to snap, how to block. So here I am, a guy who sat out for several weeks because of a head injury, participating in the act of keeping a guy who I know has a concussion out on the field." Teammates are always going to be the best at identifying concussions. They're in the huddle, and they're the most sensitive to the subtle changes in a friend's behavior on the sidelines that indicates something is wrong.

▼▼▼

Some people are trying to develop new technologies to identify concussions, some of which would take the player's motivations out of the equation. Richard Greenwald, PhD, and Simbex have developed the Head Impact Telemetry (HIT) system, where sensors inside a football helmet measure impacts in real time. These sensors could potentially alert sideline medical personnel when impacts exceed presumed concussion thresholds.

During the 2005 season, they were able to record 245,000 impacts at nine high schools and colleges. Dr. Greenwald explained the technology and their discoveries so far: "What we're seeing when a player gets a diagnosed concussion on a specific play is that when we look at the impact data, it's not necessarily the biggest hit he ever took in his life—almost invariably he took a very significant hit within forty-eight hours of the one that knocked him down. So maybe he had a concussion then, and the symptoms are still coming out.

"I think that supports several researchers' studies that say, 'The symptoms don't always appear right away, and as they appear you have to be diligent about them.' So perhaps one of the ways to be diligent about them—when they're not obvious and the player isn't reporting them—is by knowing the player's cumulative impact history over time. Then you can alert the sideline to look out for him. It's important for me to remind you that we're not trying to diagnose concussions with this system. That's left to the medical staff. But we want to give them a tool to understand when they need to look at the player more closely." This concept has potential, but it has yet to see widespread use. As Dr. Greenfield said, "It's still an expensive tool, available to Division I programs and elite high schools. It is not at a cost point to be adopted by the masses."

▼▼▼

With education and advocacy, reporting and diagnosis of concussions could substantially improve. But recognizing when a concussion has occurred is only half the battle. Concussions must be managed correctly. Studies show that it's dangerous for kids to receive secondary impacts after a concussion. But those studies don't tell us precisely where the danger ends, and they don't tell us how to convince a player not to lie about his symptoms because he's tired of sitting games out.

Even the smartest athletes lie about their symptoms. Doug Flutie, a Rhodes Scholar candidate in college, had a diagnosed concussion while playing for San Diego, but that didn't stop him from playing. "This was my best chance to start in San Diego, so I wasn't just going to hand over my position. So I didn't go too hard in practice, and I told the doctors that I felt fine. But I was having a hard time remembering the game plans, and I distinctly remember that during the next three weeks, I wasn't nearly as sharp."

Even Doug wonders if he's done any permanent damage. "In the last five years, I've noticed that things aren't as easy," he admitted to me. "It's been harder to memorize game plans, and my memory isn't quite as sharp. I hope that it is just my age, but I do wonder if it has to do with getting hit in the head so often." Parents, trainers, doctors, and coaches face an uphill battle to manage concussions properly.

CHAPTER *11*

Proper Concussion Management

I'd watch the game from the sideline, and see these guys play their hearts out and win. After the game, I'd sit on the bus thinking, "I'm a fucking pussy, standing on the sidelines in a T-shirt and jeans with a concussion, watching these guys go out and win, while I could make this a better team. We could win a state championship, but I'm not helping anybody."

Frank Rochon, 34, former high-school football player

I think the most important thing that players can do is look out for one another and play as safe as possible, understanding that when they go at a person's head, they could be creating some damage for that person. One of the things that I prided myself on was that I played the game hard, but I never tried to hurt anyone. I certainly didn't take cheap shots on guys, especially above their shoulder pads.

Harry Carson, 53, NFL Hall of Famer

The body and the head are two separate things. Below the neck if you get, like, an arm banged up, you still have another one. But you only have one head.

Ray Hill, 21, college football player

Once a concussion has been diagnosed, it isn't always exactly clear what should be done next. When I speak at schools, I usually talk about how to recognize a concussion and why it's important to rest after each one. As a favor to a friend, I spoke to the athletes at a large Massachusetts high school one week before their 2005 fall season was to begin. I was hoping that I could make a difference for a few of those athletes. I specifically emphasized that across the board, doctors advocate not returning a concussed athlete to a game if he's still suffering from symptoms.

Four months later, I attended the Harvard football post-season banquet. One of the high-school football players who'd been at my talk was sitting with his father at my table. There isn't always time for feedback after these talks, so

143

I asked him what he'd thought of it. He told me that he'd found it very interesting and logical, and that many of his teammates had, too. But then he paused and continued, "I wish that the coaches had heard it as well. You won't believe what happened. One week after your speech, we had our first game, and our middle linebacker got a bad concussion. He couldn't remember the calls and he was totally out of it. Just gone. The trainer, who's young and doesn't stand up to the coach, examined him and said he had a concussion. But I heard the coach say, 'Well, we can't put [his backup] in if we want to win.' So because he was better concussed than his backup was healthy, they left him in and he played the rest of the game."

Treatment Guidelines

In the last few years, new and better research has been pushing treatment guidelines to become more and more conservative. Once a concussion is diagnosed, the most difficult decision a trainer or coach faces is when to allow the player to return to contact. Current published guidelines indicate that this decision should be based on the severity of the concussion.

Current medical guidelines indicate that the player should not be exposed to the risk of further contact until his symptoms have cleared. If symptoms don't clear within a very short time, say within fifteen minutes of the injury, then he shouldn't return to contact activities for at least seven days, depending on the severity of his injury and how quickly his symptoms disappear.

Cantu Return-to-Play Guidelines

Grade 1	Grade 2	Grade 3
Athlete may return to play that day in select situations if clinical examination results are normal at rest and with exertion withintwenty minutes; if symptomatic, athlete may return to play in seven days if asymptomatic at rest and with exertion for seven days	Athlete may return to play in two weeks if asymptomatic at rest and with exertion for seven days	Athlete may return to play in one month if asymptomatic at rest and exertion for seven days

Source: Dr. Robert Cantu, personal correspondence

Dr. Hovda, the UCLA brain injury specialist, explained to me the logic behind basing return-to-play on the presence of symptoms. "We don't know the length of time the brain is vulnerable," he says. "But when we study humans and animals, we see that there are symptoms for as long as the (metabolic) depression exists. If we're confident that the symptoms have spontaneously alleviated, then we're pretty comfortable that the brain is back to a state where it could absorb another blow without having a devastating effect in terms of cells surviving."

But some doctors advocate that an athlete should never be returned to contact on the day of the concussion, even when symptoms have disappeared. One study of high-school athletes, known as the "Ding Study," found that even athletes who had no concussion symptoms lasting beyond fifteen minutes (according to a sideline clinical examination) still had neuropsychological deficits on computerized testing that lasted for over thirty-six hours, indicating that their brains were still vulnerable to secondary impacts during that time.[1] Another study found that continuing to play after a concussion made the symptoms worse. Of those players who returned to play on the same day, 33 percent experienced delayed onset of symptoms three hours later, while only 13 percent of kids who rested experienced new symptoms.[2]

Because it's widely known that many concussion symptoms don't appear for hours or even days, the logic behind returning players to action because they're symptom-free fifteen minutes after the injury is questionable. No objective sideline test is sensitive enough to be certain that the athlete has no symptoms, and we know that we can't rely on the athlete to always tell the truth.

A study on Army cadets at West Point clearly illustrates this point.[3] Boxing was a part of the cadets' physical education, and before the training began, all 483 cadets were given the computerized Automated Neuropsychological Assessment Metrics (ANAM), a twenty-minute battery of six subtests, in order to get a baseline score. During the boxing training, fourteen cadets were diagnosed with a mild concussion, defined by a loss of consciousness or amnesia. Those subjects were given the ANAM again one hour after their concussions, and again four days later.

For thirteen of fourteen cadets, all observable symptoms disappeared within an hour of the concussion. Yet when the cadets took the ANAM at that time, their simple reaction time was 20 percent slower than it had been before the concussion. By day four, all cadets reported no symptoms, and all had returned to physical activity. But when the test was administered again, simple reaction time had dropped even further, to 35 percent slower than the original baseline. They also still scored lower on the subtest measuring attention and concentration.

The risks caused by returning to play too soon after receiving a concussion are compounded by the simple fact that a recently concussed player is less able to defend himself.[4] [5] [6] Common post-concussion symptoms include slowed reaction time, memory impairment, and attention and concentration deficits. Split-second reaction time is often the key to avoid getting drilled in the head by one of the eleven players on the opposing team who are looking to hit you.[7]

But while science clearly indicates that immediately returning concussed players to action has major risks, indiscriminately holding out concussed athletes also has a significant downside. In a sport where most players hesitate to report concussions for fear of being pulled out of the game, automatically yanking players could make them even less likely to speak up. One research team wrote, "The easy route is to simply exclude [players with headaches] (or any injured player, for that matter) from play until their symptoms resolve. However, in our experience, such an approach quickly renders sideline physicians ineffective, because players simply stop reporting symptoms. . . . Sideline personnel who do not use their clinical judgment in these cases but instead strictly adhere to guidelines will no doubt prompt players not to report headaches or other symptoms. In the long run, this approach will probably prove more dangerous to football players than the [results] of head injuries."[8] This concern is a major reason why the Cantu guidelines still offer the option of returning players to action in the same game—it's a no-win situation, and appears to be the lesser of two evils.

The gaps in concussion treatment go far beyond determining whether to put an injured player back in the same game. The next decision concerns how long to hold the player out of action after the game. It's not as simple as strictly adhering to return-to-play guidelines, because even the authors of those guidelines admit that they're not ideal. Dr. Cantu's published guidelines correlate the length of time that a player is out of action to the concussion grade, but in the face of newer research, he now advocates that the concussion should not be graded until the symptoms have cleared. That completely changes how concussions are treated, because it eliminates the practice of predicting how long a player is expected to be out of action on the day of the injury.[9] Studies have shown that *predicting* when concussion symptoms will disappear is virtually impossible—and is in fact dangerous—because it creates expectations that the player may feel pressured to meet.

Recent evidence reveals that it can take some athletes much longer than previously believed to recover from a concussion. One recent study, using computerized neuropsychological testing, gathered and evaluated the recovery time of more than two thousand football players.[10] The study discovered that 50 percent of the athletes had not recovered after one week, and nearly 20 percent were still symptomatic after three weeks. Dr. Chae agrees with Dr. Cantu that individualized treatment is the gold standard: "The number one principle I have with brain injury treatment is individualized treatment; never generalize and always be conservative as far as protecting the brain from second injury."

But if you can't grade the concussion until symptoms have cleared, what do you tell the player? Tell him that he'll be ready to go when his brain has recovered. Period. Top doctors now advocate simply waiting until all concussion symptoms have cleared, then adding a period of rest based on how long it took the player to recover. Beware of anybody who predicts that, on the day of the injury, an athlete "will be ready to go next week."

Multiple Concussions in the Same Season

The previous guidelines are based on an athlete's suffering a single concussion. The guidelines change if the athlete suffers more than one concussion in a season. All major guidelines recommend longer periods of rest with each successive concussion, and some advocate that after the third concussion in a season, the athlete should terminate the season.

Cantu Guidelines

Severity Grade	1st Concussion	2nd Concussion	3rd Concussion
Grade 1	RTP after one week if asymptomatic	RTP one week if asympomatic for two weeks	Terminate Season
Grade 2	RTP after one week if asymptomatic for one week	Minimum of one month off sport. RTP if asymptomatic for one week. Consider termination of season	Terminate Season
Grade 3	Minimum of one month off sport. RTP if asymptomatic for one week.	Terminate Season	NA

Source: Dr. Robert Cantu, personal correspondence

While these guidelines make logical sense based on what is known about concussions, one prominent doctor has reported that the number "three" has no medical significance. Dr. Paul McCrory has written that this number is anecdotal, proposed by a Dr. Quigly in 1945 and then appearing in a major medical journal in 1952.[11]

But terminating a player's season based on the third concussion does create an interesting paradox. The Langburt incidence study found that 25 percent of high-school football players reported suffering three concussions per season, and Delaney found that 43 percent of college football players admitted the same.[12][13] The previous chapter underscores the importance of diagnosing every concussion; however, if every concussion were diagnosed, according to current guidelines, between a quarter and a half of players would not be allowed to finish the season!

Other sports aren't as concerned about rushing players back to the game. The United States Amateur Boxing guidelines for return to training or competition after concussion are far more stringent.[14]

Severity of Concussion	First Concussion	Second Concussion
A. Concussion, No LOC[15]	30-day restriction	If after (A), 90-day restriction
B. LOC < 2 minutes	90-day restriction	If after (B), 180-day restriction
C. LOC > 2 minutes	180-day restriction	If after (C), 365-day restriction

I think that concussions should be taken more seriously in football, but taking them more seriously by seeing a family physician is still no guarantee that a player will get good medical advice. A survey of 352 family physicians' general knowledge of and management practices for sports-related head injuries found that the average correct response rate was only 69.5 percent. "That's equivalent to a C-/D+ on a standard grade scale. Not that great," the study's author noted.[16] Dr. Cantu explained why these physicians have such a poor understanding of the latest information on concussions: "Most doctors who see athletes with concussions are not neurologists and neurosurgeons. The majority of them are orthopedic surgeons, pediatricians, or primary-care physicians who don't closely follow the head injury literature; they're not necessarily up on this information. In fairness, this information is evolving."

So, parents who read this book may be more up to date on the latest research than their child's physician. But by no means do I advocate not seeing a doctor. The National Athletic Trainers' Association has published a list for athletic trainers that covers the appropriate reasons to send a concussed player to a doctor or to the emergency room. Since most schools don't have trainers, this information may be more valuable in the hands of the public.

Day-of-injury referral to a physician[17]

1. Loss of consciousness on the field
2. Amnesia lasting longer than fifteen minutes
3. Deterioration of neurologic function*
4. Decreasing level of consciousness*
5. Decrease or irregularity in respirations*
6. Decrease or irregularity in pulse*
7. Increase in blood pressure
8. Unequal, dilated, or unreactive pupils*
9. Cranial nerve deficits
10. Any signs or symptoms of associated injuries, spine or skull fracture, or bleeding*
11. Mental status changes: lethargy, difficulty maintaining arousal, confusion, or agitation*
12. Seizure activity*
13. Vomiting
14. Motor deficits subsequent to initial on-field assessment
15. Sensory deficits subsequent to initial on-field assessment
16. Balance deficits subsequent to initial on-field assessment
17. Cranial nerve deficits subsequent to initial on-field assessment
18. Post-concussion symptoms that worsen
19. Additional post-concussion symptoms as compared with those on the field
20. Athlete is still symptomatic at the end of the game (especially at high-school level)

Delayed referral (after the day of injury)

1. Any of the findings in the day-of-injury referral category
2. Post-concussion symptoms worsen or do not improve over time

3. Increase in the number of post-concussion symptoms reported
4. Post-concussion symptoms begin to interfere with the athlete's daily activities (i.e., sleep disturbances or cognitive difficulties)

*Requires that the athlete be transported immediately to the nearest emergency department

Keeping Players Out

It's firmly established that a player shouldn't go back to contact if he still has symptoms. Unfortunately, we're usually at the mercy of that player to tell us whether those symptoms exist, and it's nearly impossible to know if that athlete is telling the truth.

To make matters worse, even players who believe that they're telling the truth may still be lying. Studies have documented that football players are not reliable sources of their own concussion symptoms simply because they tend to underestimate those symptoms. In the "Ding Study," players were asked to fill out a concussion symptom inventory when they performed baseline testing. The athlete scored a list of potential symptoms, such as headache and irritability, to identify if he was feeling those symptoms at the time of the test, and how severely those symptoms were affecting him.[18]

The baseline average for the group was 8.7. Thirty-six hours after a concussion, the average score jumped up to 23.3. Miraculously, six days after the concussion, the score dropped all the way down to 4.2. Now, we would expect the score to fall back to the baseline or slightly higher six days after a mild concussion. It would fall back to the baseline if the athlete had fully recovered, and it would be slightly higher if the athlete hadn't fully recovered. But the fact that it fell significantly below the baseline score is revealing. Do we really believe that six days after a concussion, an athlete feels better than he did before the concussion? Or is it more likely that, for some reason, he's trying to minimize the appearance of symptoms?

Another study by the same group of doctors found that concussed athletes usually claimed symptoms had resolved by day four. However, computerized neuropsychological testing of these athletes showed measurable cognitive deficits lingering until day seven. The authors note, "Symptom self-reporting is also likely to be influenced by the expectations of the patient and other psychological processes. In addition, some athletes are known to minimize symptoms in hopes of a faster return to the playing field, rink, or court."[19]

As long as we have to rely on players to tell us how they feel, it's our responsibility to understand why they feel pressure to minimize their symptoms. Frank Rochon was one of those players who succumbed to the pressure. As the captain of his team, he felt a responsibility to lead by example, and it got him into trouble. "I had a pretty significant head injury during my senior year," Frank told me. "We were doing a one-on-one tackling drill at camp in August, and the coach was pushing hard, yelling, 'Hit harder, hit harder!' I made a tackle on a kid named Fred Lane, who was about 6'3", 265—I was a little bigger—and we hit so hard that it made a rut in my helmet. I don't think I had a loss of consciousness or anything but I certainly don't remember a damn thing after that. It took me several hours to get back to normal. I took a day off, and then came back and kept practicing.

"The problem really manifested itself over the first couple weeks of the season. I began every practice, but after the first ding in the head, I would spend the rest of the time on the sidelines with my shoulder pads off and ice packed around my neck, trying to figure out where I was. That first little tap on the head would knock me out of it.

"The games were a completely different issue. I don't really remember any of them. I'd watch them on film and have kind of a vague remembrance of where I was, but not much actual recollection of the game itself. I played for probably six to eight weeks and yet didn't remember anything that happened on the field.

"I didn't take myself out of anything. I don't think I had the faculties to take myself out of something. I don't think I could make the rational decision to say, 'Hey I got rung up again, I just took a standing seven count—I think I need to go sit on the sideline for a few plays.' So, I just stayed out there. The only way I was coming out of the game was if my arm was broken and hanging, or my heel was facing forward. I wasn't coming out of the game on my own and saying, 'Coach, I need a couple plays off because I'm tired or my head hurts or my wrist hurts or whatever.' You just don't do that. You're not coached to do that—that's weakness.

"I remember playing a game at North Canton Hoover that was real close toward the end. I remember being on the bench, and not having a clue where I was. One of the coaches asked me, 'Are you okay, are you okay?' and I just stared at him blankly. They called the trainer over and threw a bucket of ice water on me. That brought me back a bit. Then they said, 'Get back in there and play.' I don't know if they thought it was the heat that was bugging me or what. I don't remember if we won or lost the game, but I do remember stumbling around the field after the game. The principal of the school asked me, 'Are you okay? Is everything fine?' I said something like, 'I don't have a clue where I'm at.'

"Eventually, when I felt like I just couldn't do it any more in practice, I went to the doctor. I don't really remember all the details. I do know that I had several MRI's and X-rays, and that eventually my parents and I decided that I had to sit out. I think I missed three or four games. I felt like such a wimp.

"At the end of the season, I'm looking around saying 'Crap, we're going to make the playoffs, and here I am on the sideline because of some injury that nobody can see? I feel like a complete pussy about the whole thing.' So on the bus after a game that we'd won, I turned and looked at the kid I always shared a seat with, and said, 'Hell with it, I'm playing next week. I've got to do this.' I'd probably put on 30 pounds in the four or five weeks that I didn't play. I was out of shape, but I went back out there. I couldn't have cared less what kind of damage I was doing to myself. I just wanted to go out on top; I wanted to play football."

Frank now understands what he was feeling at the time. "It's all about peer pressure. That's all it is for a kid with an injury, especially an injury you can't see. Everybody's looking at you, and it's not like you have a big knee brace on. I remember a kid on the team that year tore his knee up horribly in the preseason. He was in a wheelchair for several weeks and then crutches and a knee brace for a year. You can look at that injury and say, 'There's a reason that Eugene's not playing. Look at his knee—it's all tore up. But look at Frank over there, he's the captain of the team, he's a three-year starter, he should be an all-Ohio player this year, and he says that he's got a headache.'"

Like most of the players I spoke with who had gotten multiple concussions, Frank worries that his injuries have left a permanent mark. He said, "That's probably the worst injury that I played through and maybe the thing that did the most damage to me. It's always hard to tell if it's the concussions or just getting older, but ever since college I have headaches in the front of my head—and they're really the strangest thing, because they're not true sinus headaches, but they're definitely there. That's probably the biggest lingering issue. My decreased ability to pay attention to detail and things like that—I don't know if that's something that kind of grew into me or what.

Maybe I just have a crappy attention span, but I seem to remember having a better attention span as a high-school kid."

I asked every player I interviewed about the pressure to return from injury. They raised the same themes that are discussed in the previous chapter. However, many of them thought that the pressure grew with every day that they were on the sideline. For some, like Frank, the pressure became too much, and they felt obligated to come back before they knew that they were healed.

Part of the problem is that once a player gets injured, he's faced with the choice of "staying injured" or returning to play *every single day*. Most injuries have a prognosis; if you break your leg, you'll be out for X number of weeks. You know how long you will be out, your coaches know, and your teammates know. With a concussion, doctors try to avoid making a prognosis, so instead, the trainer, coach, and teammates have to ask the player *every day*, "Do you feel better yet?" For many, the answer to that question has less to do with how their head feels and more to do with how much longer they can answer, "No," when everyone wants to hear "Yes." How many times do you think Frank Rochon was asked that question?

But beyond the usual concerns about pressure from coaches, the injury culture, not wanting to let teammates down, and losing playing time, the athletes I interviewed also brought up three practical concerns unique to football. All three revolve around football players having a greater incentive to avoid missing games than is found in any other major team sport.

First, football has the worst ratio of games to time invested. Football players only get to play in about ten games a year. Former college player Frank Volpe explained that one of the reasons that he blew off concussions was because, "I only had ten games in the whole season. You come out of a game and you miss a week or two and that's 20 percent of your season right there. I think it means so much to players because they put in so much more pain, suffering, and all that off-season work—it's like you've invested so much into it you can't just give it up over something that seems so insignificant."

Frank hinted at the second unique aspect of football compared to major team sports—it hurts more. As former college player Brian Daigle explained, "People love to practice basketball because it's a fun sport. Although they might not admit it, nobody likes to practice football. It's tough; you suffer. You don't have the same adrenaline, the same pump that you feel on game day when you practice, so practice just wears you down. You go out there every day, pounding on the same people over and over with nothing to show for it. You're not gaining any yards; you don't have any fans yelling at you; you don't earn statistics. The only thing that you have to show for it is a beat-up body, less energy, and more pain."

The reward system is out of whack in football practice. If you make a big play in practice, not only did you just smash up your friend, but they put the ball back in the same place and tell you to do it over again.

The third motivation unique to football is that it's the only game that adults rarely play. Former Union College player Ed Lippie said it best: "Football is tougher than any other sport that I can think of. Once you're no longer good enough to play at the next level, you have no choices. Hockey players can join pickup leagues right out of college until they're in their forties and fifties. Basketball players always have a lot of opportunities to play after college, and to play competitively. But football is one of those sports that, because of the expensive equipment, because it takes eleven guys to make up one team, and because of a variety of other reasons, there's really no substitute."

The idea that a player is willing to take more risks with his body because he'll never get to play again pervaded my interviews. Many players use the "senior year" excuse, meaning that either it was their last chance to play, or that they were a leader and a lot was expected of them. The senior year excuse is in effect every year for about 25 percent of high school players, so it can lead to a lot of short-sighted decisions. Frank Volpe explained, "Let's say that you're a senior, and that this is your last chance. The last thing you want is to have some trainer telling you that you can't go out on the football field when you actually feel fine."

Psychological Consequences

As much as we'd like to think that players who rest concussions are always better off, we can't ignore the psychological consequences of forcing a player with a concussion—a guy with an invisible injury and often zero symptoms—to rest. Experts in this field note, "It is common for an athlete to report significant emotional and somatic responses to injury, including fear, anger, disbelief, rage, depression, tension, upset stomach, fatigue, insomnia, and decreased appetite," which is combined with or directly leads to anxiety, self-esteem issues, lowered pain tolerance, and introversion.[20]

What can be especially difficult about concussions is that the athlete has both a direct and an indirect psychological response to the injury. Not only might he feel terrible about not being able to play, but the part of his brain that controls emotion might be malfunctioning. It's a double whammy. Think about the young man whose entire identity is wrapped up in sports. From football, he gets meaning, purpose, self-esteem, and a social network. Take football away, and you need to replace much more than a game.

Frank Rochon got depressed. He said, "I remember being incredibly depressed in the beginning of my senior year about sitting out with a concussion. I remember not really caring that much about school, not really caring that much about anything during that period of time when I couldn't play football. Now I realize that it's pretty profound to be 17 years old and really depressed because you can't play football.

"After school, instead of going to the locker room, I would go up to the student council office and try to do my homework while everybody was changing and stretching. Eventually I would make it down to the field and stand out there for a half-hour while they were running plays or something just to try and feel involved. But I always felt like nobody really cared whether I was there or not. The rest of the team had to go on and practice and play with the idea that that I was never coming onto the field again. I went from being a captain, and feeling like an important part of the team, to being dead to the other players.

"I remember putting on weight, falling completely out of shape, and just being totally down about the whole thing. I don't even think I went to the homecoming dance that year. I didn't want to go out on weekends. I don't think I did anything. It starts to eat at you because you're so wrapped up in the game—it's your identity—that you forget that there are so many other things that are good. You forget that high-school football is just a short time in your life and it goes by and you eventually don't even talk about it any more.

"Just because you can't play, you think it will change the rest of your life—nobody likes you, you're not going to get a date with the cheerleader, you're not going to go the prom, and you're not going to get recruited to play college football. You can't let that short-term vision make you so down that it ruins your life. The only way I got out of my depression was getting back on the field, playing, and winning the title. I didn't have anybody to pull me aside and say, 'This is just a blip on the radar screen, don't worry about it.'"

How Treatment Affects Diagnosis

With all these powerful incentives for players to return to action after a concussion, I worry how increasingly conservative concussion management will affect diagnoses. As long as we need player collaboration to diagnose concussions, many athletes will consciously take into account the risk of being held out when deciding whether to mention the fact that their vision is blurry. Medical evidence and the culture of toughness are on a collision course, and I'm not sure which one will win.

It's important to remember that this is a recent phenomenon. Until ten or twenty years ago, players didn't have to worry about being held out. As the period of forced rest becomes longer and longer, we're moving into uncharted territory. My former defensive line mate, Brian Howard, said, "You can't necessarily just tell the trainer that you have a concussion, because then they'll pull you out and you won't be able to practice for at least two days. This fucks you as far as playing football goes." Brian hasn't played football in seven years. I wonder what he would have done if he thought he'd be out for two weeks.

Other Recommendations

As bleak as this chapter may seem, there are numerous ways that we can improve outcomes for athletes today. Computerized neuropsychological testing may be the most exciting opportunity. A few companies (Headminder, ANAM, Concussion Sentinel, and ImPACT) offer it for a fee.

The athlete takes about a twenty-minute computerized test at the beginning of the season. The test covers things such as memory, processing speed, and reaction time. A concussion will cause a player's scores to change. The athlete isn't allowed to return until his score returns to where it was before the injury, which would indicate that his brain function has returned to normal. These tests have been shown to be sensitive to subtle changes, and they have the advantage of producing tangible results that players and coaches can easily see for an otherwise invisible injury. The system is not foolproof, however. These tests are designed to be short and fast—which is both an advantage and a drawback. UCLA's Dr. Hovda told me, "It's sort of confusing when people say, 'Well, if I test these symptoms and they've abated, then the athlete can probably play.' Well, what if you missed a symptom that was part of a brain function that was not in an area you had tested?" Other doctors warn that developmental changes lead to improving scores, so for baseline testing of young athletes to be valid, the test would have to be performed at least every six months.[21]

One simple but radical idea that would reduce concussions is to limit the number of full-contact practices. I know that this is blasphemy to old-school coaches, but from a head injury perspective, it makes sense. The current reality is that we can't diagnose concussions. But we can prevent them by limiting exposure.

Most football players are aware that NFL teams protect their investments by ensuring that they have little to no contact in practice during the season. But few are aware that the winningest coach in the history of college football doesn't have full-contact practices either. John Gagliardi has been the head coach at Division III St. John's University in Minnesota for fifty-three seasons. Gagliardi has compiled a 432-118-11 career record using his "Winning with No's" philosophy, including no tackling in practice, no blocking sleds or dummies, and no spring practices.[22]

While his success speaks for itself, I called Coach Gagliardi to better understand why he practices this game so differently than everyone else. He explained, "We feel that the problem is not so much that we can't tackle on defense. We try to make sure that they line up in the right spot, defeat the blocking scheme, and pursue properly, and we feel that if we can get you to the ballcarrier, we don't have to prove every day that we can tackle." The players don't have practice pants; they practice in shorts. The result is that the players avoid needless injuries. "Why risk injury every day?" Gagliardi asked. "It's tough enough to beat a team with your best players, but if you get them injured. . . . We try to protect them for their sake and for our own sake. If you can prevent an injury, it's a heck of a lot simpler than to rehabilitate. We feel that we lead the world in fewest injuries, but how can we prove that? It's rare that a guy gets hurt in practice. I don't remember ever having a concussion in practice." Coach Gagliardi realizes that he has the luxury of not tackling because his players have already learned how to do that in high school. But he points out that a former St. John's player, Mike Grant, has had great success using Coach Gagliardi's methods at Eden Prairie High School in Minnesota.

Perhaps the most controversial new concept in concussion management is genetic testing. Researchers have found that head injuries are more destructive in people with a gene known as Apolipoprotein E ε4 (*APOE* ε4).[23] In some studies, possession of the gene alone doubles of the risk of Alzheimer's disease, while possession of *APOE* ε4 combined with a head injury can increase the risk of Alzheimer's disease by ten times.[24] [25] [26] Researchers believe that this risk may be caused by an interaction between *APOE* ε4 and amyloid beta.[27] This is not an isolated risk, as approximately 25 percent of the general population possesses at least one *APOE* ε4 allele.[28]

One study found evidence of this connection in a population of boxers.[29] The boxers were evaluated for chronic traumatic brain injury and graded either "probable" cases, "possible" cases, or "normal." Only 11 percent of the boxers in the study graded as "normal" or "possible" cases possessed the gene, but 50 percent of the boxers diagnosed with "probable" CTBI possessed *APOE* ε4.

Another study evaluated this phenomenon in football players.[30] Although researchers only looked at fifty-three active pro football players from one NFL team, they did find a relationship between cognitive impairment, repeated head trauma, and the *APOE* ε4 gene. The authors conclude, "Older professional football players who possessed the *APOE* ε4 allele scored lower on cognitive tests than did players without this allele or less experienced players of any genotype." The causative mechanism still remains a bit of a mystery.

Some doctors advocate incorporating a child's genetic profile into the decision of whether he should play contact sports. Dr. Daniel Amen, a clinical neuroscientist and psychiatrist, explained, "If brain injury increases the risk for Alzheimer's disease, and if you have that gene, why would we allow you to engage in sports that dramatically increase your risk for brain injury? If you have this gene, why are you going to be playing tackle football? Golf is good. Tennis is terrific. Or baseball. . . . You can have head injuries in those other things, but it's not as likely." Genetic testing would open the door to a wealth of moral, ethical, and legal problems, but it may be time to talk about it.

▼▼▼

Players face tough decisions when it comes to concussions. The best scientific research available indicates that the worst damage from concussions isn't caused by the impact itself, but by impacts to the head after the injury. The period of vulnerability is impossible to predict, and could persist for weeks. At the rate concussions occur, properly managing concussions could put one-quarter of a team on the injured reserve at any given time, and could cause those young players some serious emotional distress beyond that which is caused by the injury.

There are no easy answers here. I'm reminded of a remark made by former high-school player Nick Fisher, whose career ended with a concussion. "If you want to take care of your body, you probably won't have a place in football." I hope that's not true.

CHAPTER *12*

Facing the Challenge

Here's the problem. All of a sudden, players' bodies are bigger, stronger, and faster, so you now have players who are 6'5", 280, and can run a 4.5 40. So the physics of the hit have changed. It's a more destructive concussive hit.

Leigh Steinberg, NFL agent

Players are getting bigger, faster, more specialized, and therefore, becoming more skilled and punishing performers.[1]

David Halstead, director of the University of Tennessee
Sports Biomechanics Impact Research Lab

Would I have done it differently knowing that there are long-term issues? Probably not. The mentality of a young man is that he's invincible. In his eyes, the consequences of the physical beating that he takes are a small price to pay . . . although from this perspective, it looks like a very high price to pay.

Pete Cronan, former NFL player

The thing that no one wants to talk about is that when we were growing up, we'd play backyard football with no helmets maybe once or twice a week. Young kids today play when they're 7 years old, and you have to wonder about this accumulation of smacking and smacking. They don't know when they have a "concussion," but if it gets too rough, they probably have a way of stopping. Now you have coaches saying, "Come on! One more drill! Come on, you have to do this again and again!"

Whitey Baun, youth football coach and
former college player

To me, football's concussion crisis is like an old jigsaw puzzle. You've had it for so long that you've lost the box and forgotten what the puzzle is supposed to look like after you've put it back together. On a rainy day, you might dump the pieces from their Ziploc bag, fully intending to see it through to the end—and yet you find yourself scrambling away from it, half-finished, as soon as the sun breaks through the clouds. That's what has happened with the study of concussions in football. No one has ever seen this project through to the end, so we don't know what the completed puzzle looks like. But this book brings us one piece closer. The only reason I didn't walk away from this puzzle at some point over the last two and a half years is the sun won't break through the clouds for me. Every time I think I'm doing better, I get another week of "I-wish-I-were-dead" migraines or find that I can't get a decent night's rest. That's when I'm reminded of all the other guys who are out there struggling as well.

We're still missing pieces to this puzzle, but assembling what we do have reveals an alarming image. We know that a few kids die preventable deaths every season from second impact syndrome. We know that two former NFL players who died young under strange circumstances suffered from a degenerative brain disease caused by too many hits to the head. We know that football players who've suffered concussions are developing the same problems as people who've suffered serious head injuries, including Alzheimer's disease, depression, and cognitive impairment.

We've learned that football players are showing permanent brain damage at young ages, but we don't talk about this. The sports pages focus on those NFL players who are forced to retire prematurely due to the effects of multiple concussions, but they fail to point out that this problem also exists at the college and high-school levels. We rarely discuss the studies that show that high-school and college players with as few as two concussions can develop immediate and permanent cognitive impairment. We never package that information with the revelations that about half of the players at the high-school level and above report suffering an average of three concussions a season. Nor do we deeply consider that the consequences of concussions in children can be far worse than in adults, and can lead to permanent emotional, behavioral, and cognitive problems.

While this partial image should be attracting a lot of attention, it appears that few people are interested in pursuing the missing pieces that would complete the picture. Very little research is being done to measure precisely how much permanent brain damage is caused by concussions in football. While we're starting to look at how years of cracking skulls have affected NFL players, we have yet to undertake a single study tracking youth football players over a period of time long enough to find more definitive answers. About one in eight high-school boys plays football. It's entirely possible that a whole generation of children will soon suffer the behavioral, emotional, and cognitive problems caused by this game. It's entirely possible that those kids have laid the foundation for neurodegenerative diseases that will sap their enjoyment of life. It's also possible that the risk isn't as great as preliminary studies make it seem. But we'll never know unless we become inspired enough to find out.

Our refusal to acknowledge this health crisis means that we're missing an opportunity to prevent much of this damage right now. Just about every expert acknowledges that problems caused by concussions can be alleviated by identifying when concussions occur, and then by allowing the brain sufficient time to recover. But the reality on the field is that we've done such a poor job educating players at all levels that most can't properly identify a concussion, and few realize its negative consequences. This ignorance leaves over 90 percent of football concussions undiagnosed and untreated, and puts every one of those players at a greater risk for more permanent damage and even death.

This risk is quantitatively measurable by both the loss of life and the loss of quality of life, but perhaps the cost is best illustrated by understanding what it's like to deal with the day-to-day concerns and consequences of multiple concussions while in the prime of your life. When I began this book, my goal was to understand what was happening inside my head and what it meant for my future. I now have a pretty clear understanding of what has happened, is happening, and will happen inside my own head. But a conversation with a friend showed me that maybe I need to look outside of my own body to grasp the full impact of my head injury experiences. It might take decades before I realize that the greatest burden of a neurodegenerative disease will not be borne by me, but by the people I love and by the people who love me.

I learned this lesson from a man known to wrestling fans around the world as "Tommy Dreamer." Tom Laughlin is known throughout the business as one of the kindest, most generous, and most honorable men in wrestling. But he is also one of the craziest, and he has paid for it. In his lifetime, he has suffered thirteen documented concussions, has been knocked unconscious three times, and once had three concussions in a week.

Now that Tommy is the father of two little girls, he thinks more about the role those concussions will play in his life. But Tommy is one of the rare few who don't have to imagine his future; he stares his fears straight in the eye every day. Tommy's father has Parkinson's disease and dementia and lives with Tommy and his wife.

Tommy believes that he is already suffering from the effects of his concussions. His wife has noticed that his attention span and short-term memory are both greatly diminished. She has also noticed that he often repeats himself, telling incoherent, rambling stories that never reach a point. Last Christmas, Tommy bought and wrapped a toy for his nephew and left it under the tree on Christmas Eve. When the nephew opened the toy on Christmas morning Tommy got angry, shouting, "Man, that's what I was going to get you! Who got him that?" He didn't remember buying or wrapping the gift—but he did remember his wife looking at him as if he were crazy.

Tommy has no idea what caused his father's Parkinson's and dementia (his father played high-school football, but no one knows his concussion history), but he knows that he's at a greater risk for a similar neurological disease, and seeing his father in his condition upsets him. "He was a brilliant man, and he suffers greatly," Tommy told me. Mr. Laughlin was a superintendent of schools, a principal, and a teacher. Now he sometimes talks to people who aren't there or speaks of things that happened decades ago as if they happened yesterday. He needs help eating because his hands shake so much and help getting off the toilet when his legs lock up.

Tommy said, "The one thing that bothers me the most, and the one thing that I look into the future and say I would never want that to happen to me is when I walk into a restaurant with my family, people look at my father as if he were handicapped. They look at him as if he were emotionally disturbed, or had been burned, or had some sort of deformity. That sucks, because he's my father. If they could only see how he was . . . he'd want to show everybody the man he once was."

While Tommy will never be able to predict for certain if what is happening to his father will happen to him, he knows that he's going about fighting the odds in the wrong way. So while he still has a choice, Tommy refuses to accept that future for himself. "I want people to know me as I was, not having to be led by the hand or needing help in the bathroom. That's why I've told my wife, 'If I ever get like that, either you are going to kill me or I'll kill myself, because I don't want to be like that.' So if I ever swallow a shotgun shell because I'm all fucked up, it's because I don't want to suffer.

You heard it here first. I personally can't live my life like that." (Tommy's father passed away soon after this interview.)

▼▼▼

It is clear that there's more to football's concussion epidemic than meets the eye. At this point, I'm sure many of you who are reading this book wish that none of it were true. I'm right there with you. But the fact remains that more concussions happen in football than we're able to diagnose, and their consequences are far worse than previously known.

This information puts football at a crossroads. Either we reform football, or we try to sweep this information under the rug and hope that it goes away. I wish for the first and I fear that certain powerful groups will push for the second. But if Major League Baseball had to go before Congress simply because it didn't test for steroids, I think that this national health crisis will get the attention it is due.

At some point, we'll be forced to face this problem head on because from here it should only get worse—both on and off the field. Players are getting bigger, stronger, and faster, making the forces involved in collisions more powerful than ever. Due to gains in strength and size, the force generated by the average NFL offensive lineman has essentially doubled since 1920, and a similar trend is occurring at the lower levels of the game.[2] Therefore, even as we continue to develop new technologies and better medical treatment, we're not going to see an end to this silent epidemic.

Off the field, I expect to see long-term problems grow more pronounced. The game is not the same as it was forty years ago. Not only are players bigger, stronger, and faster, but they initiate contact differently. During the late 1960s, tackling changed from dragging a guy down to knocking him down, and the record of that change must exist in the bodies of the players. There must be a reason that Mike Webster was the first ex-NFL player to be diagnosed with CTE, and there must be a reason that, according to the NFL, no active player retired from post-concussion syndrome before 1992. This is a new game, and it has new problems.

But the situation is far from hopeless. Many of the negative consequences from concussions occur due to a lack of awareness. You can help solve these problems by being an informed activist for your family, your team, or your community. You can take enormous strides toward lowering the risks posed by concussions and make football a more positive experience for everyone involved.

I have focused on providing a comprehensive view of these injuries because it takes a certain depth of knowledge to recognize both the urgency and complexity of reform. But let me boil it down to some simple steps that we can take.

1. Improve diagnosis rates through education.

The greatest problem with a concussion may not be the injury itself, but what happens in the days and weeks after the injury. Trainers diagnosis fewer than 10 percent of the concussions that occur, so we need to find ways to identify the other 90 percent. Since trainers are only available at one out of every three schools, other people must step up and help athletes in their time of need. This role can be best filled by parents.

The first step is education. Identifying the symptoms of a concussion is not rocket science. With the state of concussion education as poor as it is today (half of college athletes don't know that concussions can have negative consequences[3]) parents should sit down with their children and explain precisely what the symptoms of a concussion are, and why it is important to tell an adult when one has occurred. Athletes learn from coaches that there is a difference between being "hurt" and being "injured." Using that framework, they will get it if a parent teaches them that a concussion *always* means they are injured, and *never* merely hurt. They should explain that an athlete is responsible for his own health and his own brain, because no one else can know exactly how he feels. And parents should let players know that they also have a responsibility to watch for these problems in their teammates. If a player notices that a teammate is experiencing concussion-like symptoms, he only does him a disservice if he doesn't alert an official, a coach, a trainer, or a parent.

With that said, parents can also play a major role in objectively diagnosing the injury. Parents have the distinct advantage of knowing their child better than anyone else. For various reasons, athletes don't always want their concussion to be diagnosed, but their behavior will reveal subtle signs of the injury, such as changes in personality and sleeping patterns. Those are often things that only parents can recognize.

2. Take a holistic approach to treatment.

Parents should take an active role in treatment as well. The best treatment involves far more than memorizing return-to-play guidelines. Most doctors are not up to date on the information provided in this book, so you shouldn't always assume that they know what is best.

Proper treatment involves an approach that emphasizes both medical and psychological concerns. The medical message is simple: an athlete should not return to action while still experiencing symptoms. But enforcing that rule can be difficult. Athletes feel pressure from coaches, teammates, and themselves to get back onto the field as soon as possible. That will often involve minimizing symptoms or lying about them. I've done it myself. Therefore, conservatively treating concussions should be combined with education and a discussion of why it is important for athletes to be honest about their symptoms.

Understanding and even embracing the unpredictable nature of these injuries is essential. Every concussion is unique, so it's both impossible and dangerous to create expectations for the athlete. While it's important to take a minimum amount of time off, with many experts recommending at least a week, many athletes will require a much longer rest—but it is impossible to predict which athlete that will be.

3. Do not rely on technology.
Everyone seems to be trying to make a buck by offering quick fixes to the concussion problem. They do not exist. Be a critical consumer. There is no reliable evidence that mouthguards have any effect on concussions. The effectiveness of helmets to prevent concussions is limited. No one has definitively proven that newer helmet designs are better than older models, but we do know that helmets wear out over time. Parents should pay attention to how long their child's helmet has been in service.

Computerized neuropsychological testing has considerable advantages, but by no means is it foolproof. Its effectiveness is limited, since it only helps that 10 percent of players who have already been diagnosed with a concussion. And while technology is wonderful, the sociologist in me knows that technological solutions are realistically available only to more affluent school districts. If two-thirds of schools don't have enough money in the budget for an athletic trainer, and if some schools now require athletes to pay to take part in sports, buying newer helmets or fancy computer programs will not be a viable option.[4]

4. Consider postponing your child's football career.
Although I'm sure youth football organizations will think I'm trying to put them out of business, the evidence points to the logical conclusion that a

shorter career is a safer career. Dr. Bennett Omalu put it very simply: "My hypothesis is that the younger you are when you start playing, and the longer you play, the higher your risk." Starting to play football at an older age solves both those problems.

5. Take responsibility.

I often hear people say, "Football players know what they're getting into." Other people believe that by presenting the correct medical information to players and warning them that concussions are dangerous, we shift the responsibility for the negative consequences of playing to the athlete. I have a hard time buying those arguments. In our society, we don't believe that young people are capable of making rational, adult decisions. (For example, you cannot be tried as an adult in our legal system until you've entered your late teens.) So, how can we expect a 14-year-old to fully grasp the complex neuroscience that explains the risk he's taking by keeping quiet after suffering a concussion? It's our responsibility as guardians to do what we can to give these young athletes a fighting chance to reach adulthood while still able to reach their full potential.

6. Be a voice of change.

Football organizations don't want to acknowledge that the concussion problem is serious enough to merit their attention. Don't accept that. The evidence for reform in football has been laid out here in a plain, straightforward manner. The debate must focus not on whether reform should occur, but how much reform there should be.

Yet change will be difficult without pressure from the grassroots level. Create that pressure. Start discussions with other parents through a booster club or simply in the stands at games. Get a group of concerned parents onboard, present a unified front, and approach the coach or trainer. State that you want the symptoms of concussions posted along with the potential outcomes of failing to report concussions (problems in school, long-term impairment, second impact syndrome, etc.). Demand that someone give a talk to the players about concussions. It can be as simple as Dr. Nichols's 1905 speech to the Harvard team that reminded the players of their responsibility to alert an adult if a teammate was acting strangely.

Expect resistance, though, because some people will see this as a way to discourage participation. Others will resist simply because they don't understand the scope of the problem. Let's face it—no one has ever put the research together in this way, so few people have this information. If the coach fails to act on your requests, approach a principal or a youth league official. Use this book as a networking and educational tool. Take this mission as far as you think you should. The power is in your hands, literally. Right now, you're holding the best concussion handbook available, so you can decide for yourself how hard you want to push this issue.

In the opening chapter, I mention that I expect to have a son someday who will want to play football. Whenever I talk about my research with people, they always ask, "Would you let your son play?" The answer is that I don't know. Nor do I know whether or not the risks of this specific game are worth it for you or for your child. My goal is simply to make sure that you base your decision on the best available information.

This information has the power to save lives and ease suffering. But it was too late to help me, and that will always be a source of great frustration. A part of me wishes that this whole thing had never happened and that I was back in the wrestling ring. But it did happen, and I'm making the best of it.

References

Chapter 1

1. De Lench, Brooke. To nineteen athletes dying young. Mom's Team Media. http://www.momsteam.com/alpha/features/editorial/seventeen_athletes.shtml (accessed August 3, 2005).
2. Filas, Lee. Coaches, players vow youth football season to go on: Parents of 12-year-old who died are in favor, league says. *Daily Herald (IL)*, October 1, 2003.
3. De Lench, Brooke. To nineteen athletes dying young. Mom's Team Media. http://www.momsteam.com/alpha/features/editorial/seventeen_athletes.shtml (accessed August 3, 2005).
4. Koch, Ed. Player's death stuns school, community. *Las Vegas Sun*, November 24, 2003.
5. ABC 7 News. Teen took two blows before fatal football game: Doctors say Snakenberg died from closed head injury. *The Denver Channel*, September 22, 2004. http://www.thedenverchannel.com/news/3751851/detail.html.
6. Schevitz, Tanya. Student dies day after football-field accident. *San Francisco Chronicle*, November 8, 2004. http://www.SFGate.com/.
7. Dabe, Christopher. Arrowhead linebacker clinging to hope. *Milwaukee Journal Sentinel*, September 22, 2005.
8. Powell J, Barber-Foss K. Traumatic brain injury in high school athletes. *JAMA* 282 (1999): 958–963.
9. Sallis RE, Jones K. Prevalence of headaches in football players. *Medicine and Science in Sports Exercise*. 32:11 (Nov 2000): 1820–1824.
10. Langburt W, Cohen B, Akhthar N, O'Neill K, Lee J. Incidence of concussion in high school football players of Ohio and Pennsylvania. *Journal of Child Neurology* 16:2 (February 2001): 83–85.
11. Edholm, Eric. Part warrior, part tragedy, Webster lived his life all the way to the end. September 27, 2002. http://www.profootballweekly.com/PFW/Commentary/Columns/2002/edholm092702.htm.
12 Associated Press. Sports Illustrated.com. http://sportsillustrated.cnn.com/2004/football/nfl/05/26/bc.fbn.pensionplan.laws.ap.
13. Omalu BI, DeKoskey ST, Minister RL, et al. Chronic traumatic encephalopathy in a National Football League player. *Neurosurgery*. 57:1 (July 2005): 128–134.

14. Guskiewicz KM, Bailes J, Marshall SW, Cantu RC. Recurrent sport-related concussion linked to clinical depression. 2003 A.C.S.M. Annual Meeting—Free Communications. San Francisco. *Medicine and Science in Sports & Exercise* 35:5 (2003): S50.

15. Guskiewicz KM, Marshall SW, Bailes JB, et al. Association between recurrent concussion and late-life cognitive impairment in retired professional football players. *Neurosurgery* 57:4 (2005): 719–726.

16. Williams, David. Press release, University of North Carolina. New study at UNC shows concussions promote dementias in retired professional football players. October 10, 2005.

17. Wilson, Duff. M.L.B. medical adviser falsifies resume. *The New York Times*, March 29, 2005.

18. Mandak, Joe. *The Associated Press*. Pathologist challenges Steelers doctor over autopsy. September 15, 2005.

19. Kaut KP, DePompei R, Kerr J, Congeni J. Reports of head injury and symptom knowledge among college athletes: Implications for assessment and educational intervention. *Clin J Sport Med* 13:4 (July 2003): 213–221.

20. Pellman EJ, Powell JW, Viano DC, et al. Concussion in professional football: Epidemiological features of game injuries and review of the literature—part 3. *Neurosurgery* 54:1 (January 2004): 81–94.

21. Pellman EJ, Viano DC, Casson IR. Concussion in professional football: Repeat injuries—Part 4. *Neurosurgery* 55:4 (October 2004): 860–876.

22. Seabrook, John. Tackling the competition. *The New Yorker*, November 18, 1997.

23. Langburt W, Cohen B, Akhthar N, O'Neill K, Lee J. Incidence of concussion in high school football players of Ohio and Pennsylvania. *Journal of Child Neurology* 16:2 (February 2001): 83–85.

24. Delaney JS, Lacroix VJ, Leclerc S, Johnston KM. Concussion among university football and soccer players. *Clin J Sport Med* 12:6 (November 2002): 331–338.

Chapter 2

1. Leiker, Ken, in collaboration with Mark Vancil. *WWE Unscripted*. New York: Simon and Schuster, 2003.

2. Ibid.

Chapter 3

1. Quality Standards Subcommittee, American Academy of Neurology. Practice parameter: The management of concussion in sports. *Neurobiology* 48 (1997): 1–5.
2. Pellman EJ, Viano DC, Tucker AM, et al. Concussion in professional football: Reconstruction of game impacts and injuries. *Neurosurgery* 53:4 (October 2003): 799–812.
3. Quality Standards Subcommittee, American Academy of Neurology. Practice parameter: The management of concussion in sports. *Neurobiology* 48 (1997): 1–5.
4. Gennarelli TA, Graham DI. Neuropathology of head injuries. *Semin Clin Neuropsychiatry* 3 (1998): 160–175.
5. Guskiewicz KM, Bruce SL, Cantu RC, et al. National Athletic Trainer's Association position statement: Management of sports–related concussion. *Journal of Athletic Training.* 39:3 (Sept 2004): 280–297.
6. Ibid.
7. Giza CG, Hovda DA. The neurometabolic cascade of concussion. *Journal of Athletic Training* 36:3 (2001): 228–235.
8. Fineman I, Giza CC, Nahed BV, Lee SM, Hovda DA. Inhibition of neocortical plasticity during development by a moderate concussive brain injury. *J Neurotrauma* 17 (2000): 739–749.
9. Ip EY, Giza CC, Griesbach GS, Hovad DA. Effects of enriched environment and fluid percussion injury on dendritic arborization within the cerebral cortex of the developing rat. *J Neurotrauma* 19 (2002): 573–585.
10. Giza CG, Hovda DA. The neurometabolic cascade of concussion. *Journal of Athletic Training* 36:3 (2001): 228–235.
11. Jenkins LW, Moszynski K, Lyeth BG, et al. Increased vulnerability of the mildly traumatized rat brain to cerebral ischemia: The use of controlled secondary ischemia as a research tool to identify common or different mechanisms contributing to mechanical and ischemic brain injury. *Brain Res* 477 (1989): 211–224. Cited in Hovda DA, et al. The neurochemical and metabolic cascade following brain injury: Moving from animal models to man. *Journal of Neurotrauma* 12:5 (1995): 903–906.
12. Giza CG, Griesbach GS, Hovda DA. Experience-dependent behavioral plasticity is disturbed following traumatic injury to the immature brain. *Behav Brain Res* 157:1 (2005): 11–22.

Chapter 4

1. Cantu, RC. Comment on Maroon JC, Lovell M, Norwig J, Podell K, Powell J, Hartl R. Cerebral concussion in athletes: Evaluation and neuropsychological testing. *Neurosurgery* 47:3 (September 2000): 659.

2. Drubach DA, Makley M, Dodd ML. Manipulation of central nervous system plasticity: A new dimension in the care of neurologically impaired patients. *Mayo Clin Proc* 79 (2004): 796–800. Citing Von Monakow C. Diachisis. In Pribham KH, ed. *Brain and Behavior I: Mood States and Mind.* Baltimore, MD: Penguin Books 1969: 27–36 and Feeney DM, Baron JC. Diachisis. *Stroke* 17 (1986): 817–830.

3. Cantu, RC. Comment on Maroon JC, Lovell M, Norwig J, Podell K, Powell J, Hartl R. Cerebral concussion in athletes: Evaluation and neuropsychological testing. *Neurosurgery* 47:3 (September 2000): 659.

4. Guskiewicz, KM, et al. Epidemiology of concussion in collegiate and high school football players. *Am J Sports Med* 28 (2000): 643–650.

5. Gerberich SG, Priest JD, Boen JR, Straub CP, Maxwell RE. Concussion incidences and severity in secondary school varsity football players. *Am J Public Health* 73 (1983): 1370–1375.

6. Zemper, ED. Relative risk of cerebral concussion in football. Paper presented at the annual meeting of the American College of Sports Medicine (Seattle, WA, June 1–5, 1999).

7. Zemper, ED. Two-year prospective study of relative risk of a second cerebral concussion. *Am J Phys Med Rehabil* 82 (2003): 653–659.

8. Guskiewicz KM, McCrea M, Cantu RC, et al. Cumulative effects associated with recurrent concussion in collegiate football players: The NCAA concussion study. *JAMA* 290:19 (November 19, 2003): 2549–2555.

9. Collins MW, Lovell MR, Iverson GL, et al. Cumulative effects of concussion in high school athletes. *Neurosurgery* 51:5 (2002): 1175–1181.

10. Gerberich SG, Priest JD, Boen JR, Straub CP, Maxwell RE. Concussion incidences and severity in secondary school varsity football players. *Am J Public Health* 73 (1983): 1370–1375.

11. Vastag B. Football brain injuries draw increased scrutiny. *JAMA* 287:4 (January 23/30, 2002): 437–439, citing Moore AH, Osteen CL, Chatziioannou AF, et al. Quantitative assessment of longitudinal metabolic changes *in vivo* after traumatic brain injury in the adult rat using FDG-MicroPET. *J Cereb Blood Flow Metab* 20 (2000): 1492–1501.

12. Giza CG, Hovda DA. The neurometabolic cascade of concussion. *Journal of Athletic Training* 36:3 (2001): 228–235.

13. Drubach DA, Makley M, Dodd ML. Manipulation of central nervous system plasticity: A new dimension in the care of neurologically impaired patients. *Mayo Clin Proc* 79 (2004): 796–800.

14. Giza CC, Griesbach GS, Hovda DA. Experience-dependent behavioral plasticity is disturbed following traumatic injury to the immature brain. *Behav Brain Res* 157:1 (February 10, 2005): 11–22.

15. Cantu RC. Second-impact syndrome: What is it? http://www.teamsof angels.org/research/head_injury_info_second_impact_syndrome.shtml.

16. Cantu RC, Voy R. Second impact syndrome: A risk in any contact sport. *The Physician and Sportsmedicine* 23:6 (1995).

17. Vastag B. Football brain injuries draw increased scrutiny. *JAMA* 287:4 (January 23/30, 2002): 437–439.

18. Dillman, Lisa and Mai Tran. Blows to head likely caused Colby's death. *Los Angeles Times*, December 7, 2001. www.momsteam.com.

19. Moore, Ann. Head injuries grim reality of athletics. WTVW, Evansville, IN. http://www.wtvw.com/.

20. Brandon Schultz news release. High school football player who sustained catastrophic brain injury settles law suit with school district. http://www.firmani.com/SIS-case/release.htm.

Chapter 5

1. Kaut KP, DePompei R, Kerr J, Congeni J. Reports of head injury and symptom knowledge among college athletes: Implications for assessment and educational intervention. *Clin J Sport Med* 13:4 (July 2003): 213–221.

2. Guskiewicz, KM, et al. Epidemiology of concussion in collegiate and high school football players. *Am J Sports Med* 28 (2000): 643–650.

3. Barth JT, Alves WM, Ryan TV, et al. Mild head injury in sports: Neuropsychological sequelae and recovery of function. In Levin HS, Eisenberg HM, Benton AL, eds. *Mild Head Injury*. New York: Oxford University Press, 1989: 257–275.

4. Guskiewicz KM, et al. Cumulative effects associated with recurrent concussion in collegiate football players: The NCAA concussion study. *JAMA* 290:19 (November 19, 2003): 2549–2555.

5. Zemper, ED. Two-year prospective study of relative risk of a second cerebral concussion. *American Journal of Physical Medicine and Rehabilitation* 82:9 (September 2003).
6. McCrea M, Kelly JP, Kluge J, Ackley B, Randolph C. Standardized assessment of concussion in football players. *Neurology* 48 (1997): 586–588.
7. Powell J, Barber-Foss K. Traumatic brain injury in high school athletes. *JAMA* 282 (1999): 958–963.
8. Langburt W, Cohen B, Akhthar N, O'Neill K, Lee J. Incidence of concussion in high school football players of Ohio and Pennsylvania. *Journal of Child Neurology* 16:2 (February 2001): 83–85.
9. Delaney JS, Lacroix VJ, Leclerc S, Johnston KM. Concussion among university football and soccer players. *Clin J Sport Med* 12:6 (November 2002): 331–338.
10. Delaney JS, Lacroix VJ, Leclerc S, Johnston KM. Concussions during the 1997 Canadian Football League season. *Clin J Sport Med* 10:1 (January 2000): 9–14.
11. Jancin, Bruce. College football players often underreport head injury symptoms to coaches and trainers. Larik Woronzoff-Dashkoff, MD. *Family Practice News*, May 15, 2001. http://findarticles.com/cf_dls/m0BJI/10_31/76004491/print.jhtml and personal correspondence.
12. Gerberich SG, Priest JD, Boen JR, Straub CP, Maxwell RE. Concussion incidences and severity in secondary school varsity football players. *Am J Public Health* 73 (1983): 1370–1375.
13. McCrea M, Hammeke T, Olsen G, Leo P, Guskiewicz K. Unreported concussion in high school football players: Implications for prevention. *Clin J Sport Med* 14:1 (January 2004): 13–17.
14. Sefton JM, Pirog K, Capitao A, et al. An examination of factors that influence knowledge and reporting of mild brain injuries in collegiate football. *Journal of Athletic Training.* 39:2. (June 2004).
15. Koh JO, Cassidy JD. *Clin J Sports Med* 14:2 (March 2004): 72–79.
16. Associated Press. Officials worry about athlete head trauma. May 20, 2004. ESPN.com. http://sports.espn.go.com/oly/news/story?id=1805836.
17. Waxman, Henry, and Jesse L. Jackson Jr. Letter to William C. Martin, Acting President of the U.S. Olympic Committee. April 21, 2004. http://www.waxman.house.gov/.
18. McCrory P, Collie A, Anderson V, Davis G. Can we manage sport related concussion in children the same as in adults? *British Journal of*

Sports Medicine 38 (2004): 516–519. Citing Ommaya AK, Goldsmith W, Thibault L. Biomechanics and neuropathology of adult and pediatric head injury. *Br J Neurosurg* 16:3 (2002): 220–242.

19. Giza CG, Hovda DA. The neurometabolic cascade of concussion. *Journal of Athletic Training.* 36:3 (2001): 228–235.

20. Field M, Collins MW, Lovell MR, Maroon J. Does age play a role in recovery from sports-related concussion? A comparison of high school and collegiate athletes. *J Pediatr* 142:5 (May 2003): 546–553.

21. Collins MW, Lovell MR, Iverson GL. Examining concussion rates and return to play in high school football players wearing newer helmet technology: A three-year prospective cohort study. *Neurosurgery* 58:2 (February 2006).

22. Lovell MR, Collins MW, Iverson GL. Grade 1 or "ding" concussions in high school athletes. *Am J Sports Med* 32:1 (Jan–Feb 2004): 47–54.

23. Cantu RC. Recurrent athletic head injury: Risks and when to retire. *Clin Sports Med* 22 (2003): 593–603.

24. Wallis, Claudia. What makes teens tick. *Time*, May 10, 2004.

25. Giza CC, Griesbach GS, Hovda DA. Experience-dependent behavioral plasticity is disturbed following traumatic injury to the immature brain. *Behav Brain Res* 157:1 (February 10, 2005): 11–22.

26. Yeoman, Barry. Lights out: Can contact sports lower your intelligence? *Discover* 24:12 (December 2004).

27. Fineman I, Giza CC, Nahed BV, Lee SM, Hovda DA. Inhibition of neocortical plasticity during development by a moderate concussive brain injury. *J Neurotrauma* 17 (2000): 739–749.

28. Ip EY, Giza CC, Griesbach GS, Hovda DA. Effects of enriched environment and fluid percussion injury on dendritic arborization within the cerebral cortex of the developing rat. *J Neurotrauma* 19 (2002): 573–585.

29. Yeoman, Barry. Lights out: Can contact sports lower your intelligence? *Discover* 24:12 (December 2004).

30. Grundl PD, Biagas KV, Kochanek PM, et al. Early cerebrovascular response to head injury in immature and mature rats. *J Neurotrauma* 11 (1994). 135–148.

31. Biagas KV, et al. Postraumatic hyperemia in immature, mature, and aged rats: Autoradiographic determination of cerebral blood flow. *J Neurotrauma* 13 (1996): 189–200.

32. McDonald JW, Johnston MV. Physiological pathophysiological roles of excitatory amino acids during central nervous system development. *Brain Res Rev* 15 (1990): 41–70.

33. McDonald JW, Silverstein FS, Johnston MV. Neurotoxicity of N-methyl-D-aspartate is markedly enhanced in developing rat central nervous system. *Brain Res* 459 (1988): 200–203.

34. Ewing-Cobbs L, Barnes M, et al. Modeling of longitudinal academic achievement scores after pediatric traumatic brain injury. *Dev Neuropyschol* 25:1–2 (2004): 107–133.

35. Hawley CA, Ward AB, Magnay AR, Long J. Outcomes following childhood head injury: A population study. *J Neurol Neurosurg Psychiatry* 75:5 (May 2004): 737–742.

36. Geraldina P, et al. Neuropyschiatric sequelae in TBI: A comparison across different age groups. *Brain Injury* 17:10 (October 2003): 835–846.

37. Bloom DR, Levin HS, Ewing-Cobbs, et al. Lifetime and novel psychiatric disorders after pediatric traumatic brain injury. *J Am Acad Child Adolesc Psychiatry* 40:5 (May 2001): 572–579.

38. Press release, University of Warwick, May 20, 2004. http://www.newsandevents.warwick.ac.uk/index.cfm?page=pressrelease&id=1912.

39. Collins MW, Grindel SH, Lovell MR, et al. Relationship between concussion and neuropsychological performance in college football players. *JAMA* 282 (1999): 964–970.

40. Ponsford J, Wilmott C, Rothwell A, et al. Cognitive and behavioral outcome following mild traumatic head injury in children. *J Head Trauma Rehabil* 14:4 (1999): 360–372.

41. Lovell M, Iverson G, Collins M, et al. Does loss of consciousness predict neuropsychological decrements after concussion? *Clin J Sport Med* 9 (1999): 193–199

42. Farmer MY, Singer HS, Mellits ED, et al. Neurobehavioral sequelae of minor head injuries in children. *Paediatr Neurosci* 13 (1987): 304–308.

43. Fay GC, Jaffe KM, Polissar NL, et al. Mild pediatric traumatic brain: A cohort study. *Arch Phys Med Rehabil* 74 (1993): 895–901.

44. Asarnow RF, Satz P, Light R, et al. The UCLA study of mild closed head injury in children and adolescents. In Broman S, Micehl ME, eds. *Traumatic Head Injury in Children*. New York: Oxford University Press, 1995.

45. Ponsford J, Willmott C, Rothwell A, et al. Impact of early intervention on outcome after mild traumatic brain injury in children. *Pediatrics* 108 (2001): 1297–1303.

Chapter 6

1. Press release. *Blazing Trails: Coming of Age in Football's Golden Era*. John Mackey with Thom Novello. Triumph Books. http://www.triumphbooks.com/BlazingTrails-press%20release.htm
2. De KJ, Twijnstra A, Leffers P. Diagnostic criteria and differential diagnosis of mild traumatic brain injury. *Brain Inj* 15 (2001): 99–106.
3. Maese, Rick. NFL neglect of Mackey belongs in the hall of shame. *Baltimore Sun*, December 27, 2005.
4. Rosso SM, Landweer EJ, Houterman M, et al. Medical and environmental risk factors for sporadic frontotemporal dementia: A retrospective case-control study. *Journal of Neurology Neurosurgery and Psychiatry* 74 (2003): 1574–1576.
5. Koponen S, Taiminen T, Portin R, et al. Axis I and II psychiatric disorders after traumatic brain injury: A 30-year follow-up study. *Am J Psychiatry* 159 (2002): 1315–1321.
6. Zhang Q, Sachdev PS. Psychotic disorder and traumatic brain injury. *Curr Psychiatry Rep* 5 (2003): 197–201.
7. Leon-Carrion J. Dementia due to head trauma: An obscure name for a clear neurocognitive syndrome. *NeuroRehabilitation* 17 (2002): 115–122.
8. Borgaro SR, Prigatano GP, Kwasnica C, Rexer JL. Cognitive and affective sequelae in complicated and uncomplicated mild traumatic brain injury. *Brain Injury* 17 (2003): 189–198.
9. Mehta KM, Ott A, Kalmijn S, et al. Head trauma and risk of dementia and Alzheimer's disease: The Rotterdam Study. *Neurology* 53 (1999): 1959–1962.
10. Van Duijn CM, Tanja TA, Haaxma R, et al. Head trauma and the risk of Alzheimer's disease. *Am J Epidemiol* 135 (1992): 775–782.
11. Schmidt ML, et al. Tau isoform profile and phosphorylation state in dementia pugilistica recapitulate Alzheimer's disease. *Acta Neurophathol (Berl)* 101:5 (May 2001): 518–524.

12. Nemetz PN, Leibson C, Naessens JM, et al. Traumatic brain injury and time to onset of Alzheimer's disease: A population-based study. *Am J Epidemiol* 149:1 (January 1999): 23–40.

13. Collins MW, Grindel SH, Lovell MR, et al. Relationship between concussion and neuropsychological performance in college football players. *JAMA* 282:10 (Sept 8, 1999): 964–970.

14. Moser RS, Schatz P. Enduring effects of concussion in youth athletes. *Arch Clin Neuropsychol* 17:1 (2002): 91–100.

15. Moser RS, Schatz P, Jordan BD. Prolonged effects of concussions in high school athletes. *Neurosurgery* 57:2 (August 2005).

16. Delaney JS, Lacroix VJ, Leclerc S, Johnston KM. Concussion among university football and soccer players. *Clin J Sport Me*d 12:6 (November 2002): 331–338.

17. Williams, David. Press release, University of North Carolina. New study at UNC shows concussions promote dementias in retired professional football players. October 10, 2005.

18. Guskiewicz KM, Marshall SW, Bailes JB, et al. Association between recurrent concussion and late-life cognitive impairment in retired professional football players *Neurosurgery* 57:4 (2005): 719–726.

19. Molgaard CA, Stanford EP, Morton DJ, et al. Epidemiology of head trauma and neurocognitive impairment in a multi-ethnic population. *Neuroepidemiology* 190:9 (1990): 233–242.

20. Ibid.

21. Yesavage JA, O'Hara R, Kraemer H, et al. Modeling the prevalence and incidence of Alzheimer's disease and mild cognitive impairment. *J Psychiatr Res* 36:5 (2002 Sep–Oct): 281–286.

22. Ibid.

23. Huang C, Wahlund L, Svensson L, et al. Cingulate cortex hypoperfusion predicts Alzheimer's disease in mild cognitive impairment. *BMC Neurology* 2:9 (2002).

24. Tervo S, Kivipelto M, Hanninen T, et al. Incidence and risk factors for mild cognitive impairment: A population-based three-year follow-up study of cognitively healthy elderly subjects. *Dement Geriatr Cogn Disord* 17:3 (2004): 196–203.

25. Larrieu S, Letenneur L, Orgogozo JM, et al. Incidence and outcome of mild cognitive impairment in a population-based prospective cohort. *Neurology* 59:10 (November 26, 2002): 1594–1599.

26. Amieva H, Letenneur L, Dartigues JF, et al. Annual rate and predictors of conversion to dementia in subjects presenting mild cognitive impairment criteria defined according to a population-based study. *Dement Geriatr Cogn Disord* 18:1 (2004): 87–93.

27. Busse A, Bischokopf J, Riedel-Heller SG, Angermeyer MC. Mild cognitive impairment: Prevalence and incidence according to different diagnostic criteria. Results of the Leipzip Longitudinal Study of the Aged (LEILA 75+) *Br J Psychiatry* 182 (May 2003): 449–454.

28. Seel RT, Kreutzer JS. Depression assessment after traumatic brain injury: An empirically based classification method. *Arch Phys Med Rehabil* 84:11 (November 2003): 1621–1628.

29. Glenn MB, et al. Depression amongst outpatients with traumatic brain injury. *Brain Inj* 15:9 (September 15, 2001): 811–818.

30. Mathias JL, Coats JL. Emotional and cognitive sequelae to mild traumatic brain injury. *J Clin Exp Neuropsychol* 21:2 (April 1999): 200–215.

31. Kreutzer JS, Seel RT, Gourley E. The prevalence and symptom rates of depression after traumatic brain injury: A comprehensive examination. *Brain Inj* 15 (2001): 563–576.

32. Holsinger T, et al. Head injury in early adulthood and the lifetime risk of depression. *Arch Gen Psychiatry* 10 (2002): 687–695.

Chapter 7

1. Pro Football Hall of Fame website. http://www. profootballhof.com/ hof/member.jsp?player_id=227.

2. Associated Press. October 3, 2002. ESPN.com. http://espn. go.com/ classic/obit/s/2002/0924/1435977.html.

3. Garber, Greg. A tormented soul. ESPN.com. January 24–28, 2005.

4. Omalu BI, DeKosky ST, Minster RL, et al. Chronic traumatic encephalopathy in a National Football League player. *Neurosurgery* 57:1 (July 2005): 128–134.

5. Roberts AH. *Brain Damage in Boxers*. London: Pitman Medical Scientific Publishing Co., 1969.

6. Jordan BD, et al. Apolipoprotein E ε4 associated with chronic traumatic brain injury in boxing. *JAMA* 278:2 (1997): 136–140.

7. Hinkebein JH, Martin TA, Callahan CD, Johnstone B. Traumatic brain injury and Alzheimer's: Deficit profile similarities and the impact of normal ageing. *Brain Injury* 17:12 (December 2003): 1035–1042.

8. Roberts AH. *Brain Damage in Boxers.* London: Pitman Medical Scientific Publishing Co., 1969.

9. Critchley M. Medical aspects of boxing, particularly from a neurological standpoint. *Br Med J* 51:5015 (February 16, 1957): 357–362.

10. Jordan BD, Matser E, Zimmerman RD, et al. Sparring and cognitive function in professional boxers. *Physician Sports Med* 24 (1996): 87–98.

11. Jordan BD, Jahre C, Hauser WA, et al. CT of 338 active professional boxers. *Radiology* 2 (1992): 181–185.

12. Jordan BD. Chronic traumatic brain injury. In *Sports-Related Concussion*, Bailes JE, Lovell MR, and Maroon JC, eds. St. Louis: Quality Medical Publishing, 1999.

13. Chen XH, Siman R, Iwata A, et al. Long-term accumulation of amyloid-β, β-secretase, presenilin-1, and caspase-3 in damaged axons following brain trauma. *American Journal of Pathology,* 165:2 (August 2004): 357–371.

14. Hamberger A, Huang YL, Zhu H, et al. Redistribution of neurofilaments and accumulation of beta-amyloid protein after brain injury by rotational acceleration of the head. *J Neurotrauma* 20:2 (February 2003): 169–178.

15. Iwata A, Chen XH, McIntosh TK, et al. Long-term accumulation of amyloid-β in axons following brain trauma without persistent upregulation of amyloid precursor protein genes. *Journal of Neuropathology and Experimental Neurology* 61:12 (December 2002): 1056–1068.

16. Uryu K, Laurer H, McIntosh T, et al. Repetitive mild brain trauma accelerates aβ deposition, lipid peroxidiation, and cognitive impairment in a transgenic mouse model of Alzheimer amyloidosis. *The Journal of Neuroscience* 22:2 (January 15, 2002): 446–454.

17. Roberts GW, Gentleman SM, Lynch A, et al. β-amyloid protein deposition in the brain after severe head injury: Implications for the pathogenesis of Alzheimer's disease. *J Neurol Neurosurg Psychiatry* 57 (1994): 419–425.

18. Schmidt ML, et al. Tau isoform profile and phosphorylation state in dementia pugilistica recapitulate Alzheimer's disease. *Acta Neurophathol (Berl)* 101:5 (May 2001): 518–524.

19. Roberts GW, Allsop D, Bruton C. The occult aftermath of boxing. *J Neurol Neurosurg Psychiatry* 53 (1990): 373–378.

20. Tokuda T, Ikeda S, Yanagisawa N, et al. Re-examination of ex-boxers' brains using immunohistochemistry with antibodies to amyloid β-protein and tau protein. *Acta Neruopathol* 82 (1991): 281–285.

21. Iwata A, Chen XH, McIntosh TK, et al. Long-term accumulation of amyloid-β in axons following brain trauma without persistent upregulation of amyloid precursor protein genes. *Journal of Neuropathology and Experimental Neurology* 61:12 (December 2002): 1056–1068.

22. Povlishock JT, Becker DP. Fate of reactive axonal swellings induced by head injury. *Laboratory Investigation* 5 (1985): 540–552.

23. Adams JH, Doyle D, Ford I, et al. Diffuse axonal injury in head injury: Definition, diagnosis, and grading. *Histopathology* 15 (1989): 49–59.

24. Iwata A, Chen XH, McIntosh TK, et al. Long-term accumulation of amyloid-β in axons following brain trauma without persistent upregulation of amyloid precursor protein genes. *Journal of Neuropathology and Experimental Neurology* 61:12 (December 2002): 1056–1068.

25. Slemmer JE, Matser DJ, De Zeeuw CI, Weber JT. Repeated mild injury causes cumulative damage to the hippocampal cells. *Brain* 125 (2002): 2699–2709.

26. Uryu K, Laurer H, McIntosh T, et al. Repetitive mild brain trauma accelerates aβ deposition, lipid peroxidiation, and cognitive impairment in a transgenic mouse model of Alzheimer amyloidosis. *The Journal of Neuroscience* 22:2 (January 15, 2002): 446–454.

27. Hof PR, Bouras C, Buee L, et al. Differential distribution of neurofibrillary tangles in the cerebral cortex of dementia pugilistica and Alzheimer's disease cases. *Acta Neuropathol* 85 (1992): 23–30.

28. Associated Press. September 13, 2005. http://msn.foxsports.com/nfl/story/4867722.

29. LaRussa, Tony. Ex-Steeler Long drank antifreeze. *Pittsburgh Tribune-Review*, January 27, 2006.

30. Greenwood, Jill King. Terry Long's death tied to football injuries. *Pittsburgh Tribune-Review*, September 14, 2005.

31. Bouchette, Ed. Surgeon disagrees with Wecht that football killed Long. *Pittsburgh Post-Gazette*, September 15, 2005.

32. Associated Press. Ex-Steeler Long drank antifreeze to commit suicide. January 26, 2006.

33. Bouchette, Ed. Surgeon disagrees with Wecht that football killed Long. *Pittsburgh Post-Gazette*, September 15, 2005.

34. Associated Press. Ex-Steeler Long drank antifreeze to commit suicide. January 26, 2006.

Chapter 8

1. Barrow, Matthew. Brain injuries draw debate: Concern arises over diagnosing concussion such as the one suffered by 49er Jimmy Williams. *Sacramento Bee*, October 17, 2004. http://www.sacbee.com/content/sports/story/111223675p-12040043c.html.

2. McKinley, James C. Jr. A perplexing foe takes an awful toll. *New York Times*, May 11, 2000.

3. Pellman, Elliott. Interviewed by *Inside the NFL*, HBO Sports, December 10, 2003.

4. Ibid.

5. Ibid.

6. Ibid.

7. Seel RT, Kreutzer JS. Depression assessment after traumatic brain injury: An empirically based classification method. *Arch Phys Med Rehabil* 84:11 (November 2003): 1621–1628.

8. Glenn MB, et al. Depression amongst outpatients with traumatic brain injury. *Brain Inj* 15:9 (Sep 2001): 811–818.

9. Mathias JL, Coats JL. Emotional and cognitive sequelae to mild traumatic brain injury. *J Clin Exp Neuropsychol* 21:2 (April 1999): 200–215.

10. Pellman, EJ. Background on the National Football League's research on concussion in professional football. *Neurosurgery* 53:4 (October 2003).

11. Ibid.

12. Dvorchak, Robert. Steelers doctor says concluding football led to Long's demise is bad science. *Pittsburgh Post-Gazette*, September 16, 2005.

13. Borzi, Pat. Favre's concussion adds to the Packer's woes. *The New York Times*, October 4, 2004.

14. Reuters. NFL notebook. *Taipei Times*, September 14, 2003. http://www.taipeitimes.com/News/sport/archives/2003/09/14/2003067882/print.

15. Goheen, Kevin. Associated Press. Victory Sunday is crucial. *Cincinnati Post*, November 30, 2004. http://www.cincypost.com/2004/11/30/bengnotes11–30–2004.html.

16. Ibid.

17. Pittsburgh Steelers press conference. October 5, 2004. www.steelers.com.

18. Gerheim, Tim. Audibles at the line: Week 11. November 21, 2005. www.footballoutsiders.com.

19. Trotter, Jim. A softer, gentler Schottenheimer? *The San Diego Union-Tribune*, November 1, 2004.

20. Sullivan, Tim. Long-term health of Drew Brees more important than the next game. *The San Diego Union-Tribune*, September 20, 2004.

21. Associated Press. Brees expects to start despite concussion. September 20, 2004.

22. Pellman EJ, Viano DC, Casson IR. Concussion in professional football: Injuries involving 7 or more days out. Part 5. *Neurosurgery* 55:5 (November 2004): 1100–1119.

23. Associated Press. Brees expects to start despite concussion. September 20, 2004.

24. Sullivan, Tim. Long-term health of Drew Brees more important than the next game. *The San Diego Union-Tribune*, September 20, 2004.

25. Associated Press. Jets lost Chrebet for the rest of season. http://www.msnbc.com/news/992827.asp?cp1=1. November 12, 2003.

26. Jets Confidential Staff. New York Jets team report, November 6, 2003. http://jets.theinsiders.com/2/198360.html.

27. NFL.com wire reports. Chrebet to miss remainder of the season. November 12, 2003. http://www.nfl.com/teams/story/NYJ/6826352.

28. Interview, Anthony Loscalzo, March 2004.

29. Associated Press. Jets lost Chrebet for the rest of season. http://www.msnbc.com/news/992827.asp?cp1=1. November 12, 2003.

30. Jets Confidential Staff. New York Jets team report, November 6, 2003. http://jets.theinsiders.com/2/198360.html.

31. Ibid.

32. Associated Press. Jets lost Chrebet for the rest of season. http://www.msnbc.com/news/992827.asp?cp1=1. November 12, 2003.

33. Associated Press. Chrebet out for season with post-concussion syndrome. November 13, 2003. *Boston Herald*. http://patriots.bostonherald.com/otherNFL/otherNFL.bg?articleid=129&format=text.

34. Giza CG, Hovda DA. The neurometabolic cascade of concussion. *Journal of Athletic Training* 36:3 (2001): 228–235.

35. Jets Confidential Staff. New York Jets team report, November 15, 2003. http://jets.theinsiders.com/2/201923.html.

36. Cimini, Rich. Chrebet a real head case. *New York Daily News*, November 6, 2003. http://www.nydailynews.com/sports/football/v-pfriendly/story/134137p-119550c.html.

37. Jets Confidential Staff. New York Jets team report, November 6, 2003. http://jets.theinsiders.com/2/198360.html.

38. Wojtys EM, Hovda D, Landry G, Boland A, Lovell M, McCrea M, Minkoff J. Concussion in sports, from the AOSSM Concussion Workshop Group, Rosemont IL. *The American Journal of Sports Medicine* 27:5 (1999).

39. Jets Confidential Staff. New York Jets team report, November 15, 2003. http://jets.theinsiders.com/2/201923.html.

40. Cimini, Rich. Chrebet a real head case. *New York Daily News*, November 6, 2003. http://www.nydailynews.com/sports/football/v-pfriendly/story/134137p-119550c.html.

41. Pellman EJ, Viano DC, Casson IR. Concussion in professional football: Injuries involving 7 or more days out. Part 5. *Neurosurgery* 55:5 (November 2004): 1100–1119.

42. Wojtys EM, Hovda D, Landry G, Boland A, Lovell M, McCrea M, Minkoff J. Concussion in sports, from the AOSSM Concussion Workshop Group, Rosemont IL. *The American Journal of Sports Medicine* 27:5 (1999): 684.

43. Berger, Ken. Knockout blow for Chrebet. *Newsday*, November 8, 2005.

44. Associated Press. Injured New York Jets receiver Wayne Chrebet uncertain about future. December 16, 2003.

45. Cimini, Rich. Jets give Chrebet concussion clause. *New York Daily News*, March 31, 2004.

46. Berger, Ken. Chrebet agrees to re-work deal. Newsday.com, April 1, 2004.

47. Berger, Ken. Knockout blow for Chrebet. *Newsday*, November 8, 2005.

48. Adelson, Andrea. Jets receiver Wayne Chrebet retires. *Associated Press*. Forbes.com. June 2, 2006.

49. Pennington, Bill. A sports turnaround: The team doctors now pay the team. *New York Times*, May 18, 2004.

50. Calandrillo, Steve P. Sports medicine conflicts: Team physicians vs. athlete patients. *St Louis U. L.J.* 50 (2006) 185–210. http://www.law.washington.edu/Faculty/Calandrillo/Publications/Sports%20Medicine%20Conflicts%20(PDF).pdf.

51. Wilson, Duff. M.L.B. medical adviser falsifies resume. *The New York Times*, March 29, 2005.

52. ESPN.com. ESPN.com's steroid hearing scorecard. March 17, 2005.

53. Milbank, Dana. Nobody sings in this 5th Amendment stretch. *Washington Post*, March 18, 2005.

54. Wilson, Duff. M.L.B. medical adviser falsifies resume. *The New York Times*, March 29, 2005.

55. Quoted from William Sherman, Growing nightmare of steroid abuse: Athletes' cocktail big in nation's gyms. *New York Daily News*, July 28, 2002. In McCloskey, John and Julian Bailes, M.D. *When Winning Costs Too Much: Steroids, Supplements, and Scandal in Today's Sports.* Lanham, MD: Taylor Trade Publishing, 2005: 38.

56. Wilson, Duff. M.L.B. medical adviser falsifies resume. *The New York Times*, March 29, 2005.

57. Ibid.

58. Thomsen, Sara. Favre's concussion raises awareness in school athletes. WBAY TV, October 5, 2004

59. Pellman EJ, Viano DC, Casson IR. Concussion in professional football: Repeat injuries—Part 4. *Neurosurgery* 55:4 (October 2004): 860–876.

60. Pellman EJ, Lovell MR, Viano DC. Concussion in professional football: Neuropsychological testing—Part 6. *Neurosurgery* 55:6 (December 2004): 1290–1305.

61. *The Christian Science Monitor*. NFL introduces new way for kids to play. May 3, 2000.

62. Ibid.

63. Scott Lancaster biography. http://www.fairplaytoday.com/exec/fairplay/about.cfm?publicationID=64.

64. De Armas, Leigh. Catch 'em young. *Orlando Weekly*, June 2, 2005. http://www.orlandoweekly.com/features/story.asp?id=4756 (accessed April 27, 2006).

65. Ibid.

66. Keating, Peter. NFL won't bite on dentist's concussion device. *ESPN The Magazine*, February 13, 2006.

67. Ibid.

68. Ward, Sandy. National Athletic Trainers' Association. Personal correspondence. June 23, 2004.

Chapter 9

1. Garber, Greg. NFL players in harm's way. ESPN.com. January 25, 2004. http://sports.espn.go.com/espn/print?id=1718306&type =story.

2. Pellman EJ, Viano DC, Tucker AM, et al. Concussion in professional football: Reconstruction of game impacts and injuries. *Neurosurgery* 53:4 (2003): 799–814.

3. Ibid.

4. Halstead PD, Alexander CF, Cook EM, Drew RC. Historical evolution of football headgear. Unpublished, given to author through personal correspondence.

5. www.helmethut.com.

6. Lambert, Craig. First and 100: Harvard Stadium, with its storied past, is football's edifice rex. *Harvard Magazine* (September–October 2003). Chronology by John Bethell.

7. Maroon JC, et. al. Cerebral concussion in athletes: Evaluation and neuropsychological testing. *Neurosurgery* 47 (2000): 659–672.

8. Lambert, Craig. First and 100: Harvard Stadium, with its storied past, is football's edifice rex. *Harvard Magazine* (September–October 2003). Chronology by John Bethell.

9. Ibid.

10. Ibid.

11. Ibid.

12. Halstead PD, Alexander CF, Cook EM, Drew RC. Historical evolution of football headgear. Unpublished, given to author through personal correspondence.

13. National Center for Catastrophic Sport Injury Research. *Annual Survey of Football Injury Research*. 1931–2002.

14. Mueller, O. Catastrophic head injuries in high school and collegiate sports. *Journal of Athletic Training* 36:3 (2001): 312–315.

15. Ibid.

16. Ibid.

17. Halstead PD, Alexander CF, Cook EM, Drew RC. Historical evolution of football headgear. Unpublished, given to author through personal correspondence

18. Heck JF. The incidence of spearing during a high school's 1975 and 1990 football seasons. *J Athl Train* 31 (1996): 31–37.

19. Heck JF, Clarke KS, Peterson TR, et al. National Athletic Trainers' Association position statement: Head-down contact and spearing in tackle football. *J Athl Training* 39:1 (Jan–Mar 2004): 101–111.

20. Pellman EJ, Viano DC, Tucker AM, et al. Concussion in professional football: Reconstruction of game impacts and injuries. *Neurosurgery* 53:4 (2003): 799–814.

21. Ibid.

22. Ibid.

23. Ibid.

24. Kahn, Chris. Football hits, car crashes have similar impacts on skull. *The Ithaca Journal*, January 5, 2004. www.theithacajournal.com/news/stories/20040105/localnews/166892.html.

25. Garber, Greg. NFL players in harm's way. ESPN.com. January 25, 2004. http://sports.espn.go.com/espn/print?id=1718306&type =story.

26. 2002 NCAA Football Rules and Interpretations. http://www.ncaa.org/library/rules/2002/2002_football_rules.pdf.

27. National Collegiate Athletic Association. *2001 Consolidated NCAA Foul Report*. Indianapolis, IN: National Collegiate Athletic Association, 2002.

28. Heck JF, Clarke KS, Peterson TR, et al. National Athletic Trainers' Association position statement: Head-down contact and spearing in tackle football. *J Athl Training*. 2004 Jan–Mar; 39(1): 101–111.

29. 2005 Consolidated NCAA Penalty Report. Major Division 1 Football.

30. Myers TJ, Yoganandan N, Sances A Jr, et al. Energy absorption characteristics of football helmets under low and high rates of loading. *Biomed Mater Eng* 3:1 (Spring 1993): 15–24.

31. Halstead PD, Alexander CF, Cook EM, Drew RC. Historical evolution of football headgear. Unpublished, given to author through personal correspondence.

32. McCrory P, Collie A, Anderson V, Davis G. Can we manage sport related concussion in children the same as in adults? *Bj J Sports Med* 38 (2004): 516–519.

33. Timko, Steve. Skier praises helmet's protection. *Reno Gazette Journal*, January 9, 2005. http://www.rgj.com/news/printstory.php?id=89402.

34. Pellman EJ, Viano DC, Tucker AM, et al. Concussion in professional football: Reconstruction of game impacts and injuries. *Neurosurgery* 53:4 (2003): 799–814.

35. Halstead PD. Performance testing updates in head, face, and eye protection. *Journal of Athletic Training* 36:3 (2001): 322–327.

36. Halstead PD, Alexander CF, Cook EM, Drew RC. Historical evolution of football headgear. Unpublished, given to author through personal correspondence.

37. Levy ML, Ozgur BM, Berry CB, et al. Birth and evolution of the football helmet. *Neurosurgery* 55:3 (September 2004): 656–652.

38. Ommaya AK, Gennarelli TA. Cerebral concussion and traumatic unconsciousness: Correlation of experimental and clinical observations on blunt head injuries. *Brain* 97 (1974): 633–654.

39. Riddell Revolution website. http://www.riddell1.com/index.php.

40. Schutt DNA helmet fact sheet. www.schuttdna.com.

41. Glazer, Jay. NFL players to be offered Revolution-ary helmet. CBSSportsline.com. March 4, 2002. http:cbs.sportsline. com/b/page /press box/0,1328,5085894,00.html.

42. NOCSAE. *Impact Newsletter.* Summer 2003.

43. Pellman EJ, Viano DC, Tucker AM, et al. Concussion in professional football: Reconstruction of game impacts and injuries. *Neurosurgery* 53:4 (2003): 799–814.

44. Pellman EJ, Viano DC, Tucker AM, et al. Concussion in professional football: Reconstruction of game impacts and injuries—Part 2. *Neurosurgery* 53:6 (2003): 1328–1341.

45. Schutt press release. Military technology hits the gridiron head-on this bowl season. December 26, 2003.

46. Dennis, Jan. Associated Press. New football helmet brings military technology to prevent injury on playing field. December 2, 2003.

47. Raquel O. Rodriguez and Jose L. Rodriguez vs. Riddell Sports, Inc., et al. In the United States Court of Appeals for the Fifth Circuit. Case 99–40680. http://www.ca5.uscourts.gov/opinions/pub /99/ 99–40 680-cv0.htm.

48. Collins M, Lovell MR, Iverson GL, Ide T, Maroon J. Examining concussion rates and return to play in high school football players wearing newer helmet technology: A three-year prospective cohort study. *Neurosurgergy* 58:2: 275–286.

49. Dr. Ken. Helmet evolution: Safety first. Helmethut.com.http://www. helmethut.com/Dr.Ken1.html (accessed February 20, 2004).

50. Sporting Goods Business. Russell Corporation acquires Bike Athletic Company. January 31, 2003. http://www.sgblink.com/sportinggoods business/headlines/article_display.jsp?vnu_content_1807319.

51. Newsday. New football helmets under scrutiny by NFL. http://www. sportsandlawnews.com/archive/Articles%202000/NFLHemits.htm (*sic*).

Chapter 10

1. Smith, Ronald A., Ed. *Big-Time Football at Harvard, 1905: The Diary of Coach Bill Reid*. Urbana, IL: University of Illinois Press, 1994.
2. Ibid, p. 289.
3. Ibid, p. 289.
4. Ibid, p. 297.
5. Ibid, p. 303.
6. Ibid, p. 304.
7. Ibid, p. 189.
8. Larik Woronzoff-Dashkoff, MD. Personal correspondence.
9. Ward, Sandy. National Athletic Trainers' Association. Personal correspondence. June 23, 2004,
10. Tonino MP, Bollier MJ. Medical supervision of high school football in Chicago: Does inadequate staffing compromise healthcare? *The Physician and Sportsmedicine* 32:2 (February 2004).
11. Brady Merchant.
12. Delaney JS, Lacroix VJ, Leclerc SL, Johnston KM. Concussions among university football and soccer players. *Clinical Journal of Sports Medicine*. 12:6 (2002) 331–338.
13. Sallis RE, Jones K. Prevalence of headaches in football players. *Med Sci Sports Exerc* 32:11 (2000): 1820–1824.
14. McCrea M, Hammeke T, Olsen G, Leo P, Guskiewicz K. Unreported concussion in high school football players: Implications for prevention. *Clin J Sport Med* 14:1 (Jan 2004): 13–17.
15. Sefton JM, Pirog K, Capitao A, et al. An examination of factors that influence knowledge and reporting of mild brain injuries in collegiate football. *Journal of Athletic Training* 39:2 (June 2004) S52–53.
16. Ibid.
17. Ibid.
18. Lambert, Craig. The marketplace of perceptions. *Harvard Magazine* (March–April 2006): 50–57.
19. McCrea M, Kelly JP, Randolph C, Cisler R, Berger L. Immediate neurocognitive effects of concussion. *Neurosurgery* 50:5 (May 2002): 1032–1042.
20. Ibid.

21. Cantu R. Posttraumatic retrograde and anterograde amnesia: Pathophysiology and implication in grading and safe return to play. *Journal of Athletic Training* 36:3 (2001): 244–248.
22. Cantu RC. Comment on Pellman EJ, Viano DC, Casson IR, et al. Concussion in professional football: Repeat injuries—Part 4. *Neurosurgery* 55:4 (October 2004): 860–875.
23. McCrea M, Hammeke T, Olsen G, Leo P, Guskiewicz K. Unreported concussion in high school football players: Implications for prevention. *Clin J Sport Med* 14:1 (Jan 2004): 13–17.
24. Notebaert AJ, Guskiewicz KM. Current trends in athletic training practice for concussion assessment and management. *Journal of Athletic Training* 40:4 (2005): 320–325.
25. Liggett GM, Madison JB, Nitzkin JL, et al. Football-related spinal cord injuries among high school players—Louisiana 1989. *MMWR* 39 (1990): 586–587.
26. Louisiana Sports Medicine and Safety Advisory Council. Safe tackling: A training video. Louisiana Office of Public Health, Disability Prevention Program, 1991.
27. Lawrence DW, Stewart GW, Christy DM, et al. High school football-related cervical spinal cord injuries in Louisiana—The athlete's perspective. *J La State Med Soc* 149:1 (1997): 27–31.
28. Ibid.
29. Smith, Ronald A., Ed. *Big-Time Football at Harvard, 1905: The Diary of Coach Bill Reid*. Urbana, IL: University of Illinois Press, 1994. p 189.

Chapter 11

1. Lovell MR, et al. Grade 1 or "ding" concussions in high school athletes. *Am J Sports Med* 32:1 (Jan–Feb 2004): 47–54.
2. Guskiewicz KM, McCrea M, Marshall SW, et al. Cumulative effects of recurrent concussion in collegiate football players: The NCAA concussion study. *JAMA* 290:19 (November 19, 2003): 2549–2555.
3. Warden DL, et al. Persistent prolongation of simple reaction time in sports concussion. *Neurology* 57 (2001): 524–526.
4. Ibid.
5. Lovell MR, et al. Grade 1 or "ding" concussion in high school athletes. *Sports Med* 32:1 (Jan–Feb 2004): 47–54.

6. Guskiewicz KM, et al. Postural stability and neuropsychological deficits after concussion in collegiate athletes. *Journal of Athletic Training* 36:3 (2001): 263–273.

7. Giza CG, Hovda DA. The neurometabolic cascade of concussion. *Journal of Athletic Training.* 36:3 (2001): 228–235.

8. Sallis RE, Jones K. Prevalence of headaches in football players. *Medicine and Science in Sports Exercise.* 32:11 (Nov 2000): 1820–1824.

9. Cantu RC. Comment on Pellman EJ, Viano DC, Casson IR, et al. Concussion in professional football: Repeat injuries—Part 4. *Neurosurgery* 55:4 (October 2004): 860–875.

10. Collins M, Lovell MR, Iverson GL, Ide T, Maroon J. Examining concussion rates and return to play in high school football players wearing newer helmet technology: A three-year prospective cohort study. *Neurosurgergy* 58:2 (2006): 275–286.

11. McCrory PR. When to retire after concussion. *Br J Sports Med* 35:6 (Dec 2001): 380–382.

12. Delaney JS, Lacroix VJ, Leclerc S, Johnston KM. Concussion among university football and soccer players. *Clin J Sport Med* 12:6 (Nov 2002): 331–338.

13. Langburt W, Cohen B, Akhthar N, O'Neill K, Lee J. Incidence of concussion in high school football players of Ohio and Pennsyvania. *Journal of Child Neurology* 16:2 (February 2001): 83–85.

14. 1993–1995 United States Amateur Boxing, Inc. Official Rules, pp 29–31. From Cantu RC, Voy R. Second impact syndrome: A risk in any contact sport. *The Physician and Sportsmedicine* 23:6 (1995).

15. Three standing eight counts in one round or four in a bout, or the boxer receives a stunning head blow and demonstrates a lack of normal responses whether knocked out or standing.

16. Jancin, Bruce. Family physicians score D+ on sports concussion knowledge. *Family Practice News,* May 15, 2001. http://www.findarticles.com/cf_dls/m0BJI/10_31/76004490/p1/article.jhtml.

17. Guskiewicz KM, Bruce SL, Cantu RC, et al. National Trainers' Association position statement: Management of sports-related concussion. *Journal of Athletic Training* 39:3 (2004): 280–297.

18. Lovell MR, et al. Grade 1 or "ding" concussion in high school athletes. *Am Sports Med* 32:1.(Jan–Feb 2004): 47–54.

19. Lovell MR, et al. Recovery from mild concussion in high school athletes. *J Neurosurgery* 98 (2003): 296–301.

20. Putukian M, Echemendia RJ. Psychological aspects of serious head injury in the competitive athlete. *Clin Sports Med* 22 (2003): 617–630.

21. McCrory P, Collie A, Anderson V, Davis G. Can we manage sport related concussion in children the same as in adults? *Br J Sports Med* 38 (2004): 516–519.

22. http://www.gojohnnies.com/football/jg.htm.

23. Teasdale GM, Nicoll JA, Murray G, Fiddes M. Association of apolipo-protein E polymorphism with outcome after head injury. *The Lancet* 350 (October 11, 1997): 1069–1071.

24. Mayeux R, Ottman R, Maestre G, et al. Synergistic effects of traumatic head injury and apolipoprotein-ε4 in patients with Alzheimer's disease. *Neurology* 45 (1995): 555–557.

25. Tang MX, Maestre G, Tsai WY, et al. Effect of age, ethnicity, and head injury on the association between APOE genotypes and Alzheimer's disease. *Ann NY Acad Sci* 802 (1996): 6–15.

26. Corder EH, Saunders AM, Strittmater WJ, et al. Gen does of apolipoprotien E type 4 allele and the risk of Alzheimer's disease in late onset families. *Science* 261 (1993): 921–923. In Jordan BD, et al. Apolipoprotein E ε4 associated with chronic traumatic brain injury in boxing. *JAMA* 278:2 (1997): 136–140.

27. Hartman RE, Laurer H, Longhi L, et al. Apolipoprotein E4 influences amyloid deposition but not cell loss after traumatic brain injury in a mouse model of Alzheimer's disease. *The Journal of Neuroscience.* 22:23 (December 2002): 10083–10087.

28. Kutner KC, et al. Lower cognitive performance of older football players possessing apolipoprotein E ε4. *Neurosurgery* 47:3 (2000): 651–658.

29. Jordan BD, et al. Apolipoprotein E ε4 associated with chronic traumatic brain injury in boxing. *JAMA* 278:2 (1997): 136–140.

30. Kutner KC, et al. Lower cognitive performance of older football players possessing apolipoprotein E ε4. *Neurosurgery* 47:3 (2000): 651–658.

Chapter 12

1. Halstead PD, Alexander CF, Cook EM, Drew RC. Historical evolution of football headgear. Unpublished, given to author through personal correspondence.

2. Gay, Timothy. *Football Physics.* Emmaus, PA: Rodale, 2004.